'Bid the Sickness Cease'

'Bid the Sickness Cease'

DISEASE IN THE HISTORY
OF BLACK AFRICA

Oliver Ransford

JOHN MURRAY

© Oliver Ransford 1983

First published 1983
by John Murray (Publishers) Ltd
50 Albemarle Street, London W1X 4BD

Typeset by Inforum Ltd, Portsmouth
Printed and bound in Great Britain by
The Pitman Press, Bath

British Library Cataloguing in Publication Data
Ransford, Oliver
'Bid the sickness cease'
1. Environmentally induced diseases
I. Title
616'.00960   RB152
ISBN 0-7195-3986-2

Contents

Illustrations

ACKNOWLEDGEMENTS
Nos. 1, 2, 3, by courtesy of the London School of Hygiene and
Tropical Medicine. Nos. 4, 5, 6, 7, 8, 9, 10, by courtesy of the
Wellcome Trustees

Acknowledgements

I RECEIVED A great deal of help from colleagues and friends while writing this book. Particular thanks must go to two of them; Mr John R. Murray, whose assistance in putting the book together was, as always, far more than an author is entitled to expect from his publisher; and Dr C.J. Hackett who went far beyond the bounds of friendship by advising me most generously on many problems I encountered. I must stress, however, that he bears no responsibility for the statements made and conclusions reached.

It is a pleasure too, to record the specialist advice provided to me by colleagues from many parts of the world, notably Dr Norris Baker, Professor C.G. Bruce-Chwatt, Mr R. Borland, Professor D. Bradley, Dr A.J. Duggan, Dr Catherine Elliot, Professor M. Gelfand, Professor M.S.R. Hutt, Dr Alan Mills, Mr A.O. Ransford, Professor R.S. Roberts, Professor Fraser Ross and Dr R. Schram.

The staffs of the Bulawayo Public Library, the National Free Library of Zimbabwe and the Libraries of the University of Zimbabwe and of Groote Schuur Hospital were helpful to me in every way possible, and I am particularly indebted to Mrs A. Milne and Mrs G. Murphy for obtaining copies of rare articles bearing on my subject. Mrs Maud Webber kept me supplied with writing material when it ran short in beleagured Rhodesia, Miss Susan Hendrie carried the manuscript safely to London, my two daughters, Carol and Charlotte, assisted my wife in typing the preliminary text, while Mrs H.M. Grove and Mrs G. Zachariades dealt with the final version. Mr J. Gibson kindly read the proofs.

Several institutions assisted my research, including that remarkable establishment the Wellcome Museum of Medical Science, the Ciba Foundation, the Medical Division of the Longman Group in Zimbabwe, and the editors of *World Health*, the organ of the World Health Organisation.

My greatest debt of gratitude is again owed to my wife. She shared many journeys with me through tropical Africa and assisted at every stage in the preparation of this book, so it is very fitting that it be dedicated to her.

To My Wife

Africans began to venture from their villages, either to escape from slavers and the inter-tribal wars they fostered, or to trade peacefully with the white newcomers on the coast. These travellers carried with them their own pathogenic organisms to communities which possessed little natural protection against them, while they themselves became infected by diseases to which they possessed no immunity.

The period of encounter between Africans and foreigners continued for over four centuries. But even during this time the contact was only minimal because European activity was hindered by tropical diseases, and also because of the Europeans' natural disinclination to venture among the dangers of the unknown interior. Accordingly neither the old African ethos nor the incidence of sickness among Africans greatly changed.

However a new destabilising phase in Afro-European relationship developed during the late 1870s following the recognition of the therapeutic value of quinine in warding off malaria, the most dangerous of all tropical diseases. From then on increasing numbers of white explorers and entrepreneurs began to move about Africa in relative security; contact with its peoples increased and the pattern of African sickness changed. Whereas a pre-contact morbidity map would have shown small scattered foci of endemic disease* throughout the continent, now the map began to be marked by the spread of epidemic sickness to regions where they were highly dangerous to virgin communities which lacked any immunity to them.

---

* The term endemic applies to diseases which are always present in one particular area; these infections appear continuously in the population of that locality. When the diseases extend beyond their original borders they are termed epidemic. Epidemics affect large numbers of people at one time. Population movement may initiate epidemics but so do natural causes. Thus malaria may be endemic in marshy country, but becomes epidemic after heavy rains when it spreads to outside communities lacking recent experience of it. The illnesses which result are likely to be severe. When epidemics spread to another continent they are termed pandemics.

It was at this stage, during the early 1880s, that the European powers entered into a policy of 'paper-annexation' of the African continent. Statesmen in Berlin, Paris, London, Lisbon and Brussels joined each other in tracing artificial frontier lines across the map of Africa. These lines indicated their respective claims to its territory, although no effective occupation of the territories could be undertaken immediately.

The third phase, the conquest of Africa, followed quickly on the paper-partition of the continent. By 1890 the European powers were effectively established in most of Black Africa. The fourth phase in the recent history of the continent was one of consolidation by the colonial powers. It lasted until the 1960s when European influence faded and the old colonies, protectorates and mandates gained their independence.

The vital years of 1885–1930 were ones of epidemiological disaster for Africa and are studied in detail in chapter five. Before this, in the first chapter I have attempted to provide an account of the African life-style before 1885, a life-style which persists in many regions today. In chapter two I have emphasised the importance of minute animal parasites as causes of the diseases most prevalent in Africa. The three chapters that follow deal particularly with medical events which led to the European conquest of the continent and deal with the conquest itself, while the next seven provide accounts of the most serious of the African diseases. In them occasional diversions have been made to take note of earlier European reactions to tropical illnesses, since these responses were relevant to the general attack mounted on them during the present century. The final chapter concerns the new approach to the medical problems of the continent which promises to provide full health for all its people by the year two thousand.

The burst of scientific discovery, which coincided with the stabilisation of Middle Africa under white rule and the campaigns by western medical men to eradicate tropical disease from the continent, proceeded so successfully that by the middle of the 1960s complete victory against malaria and the other banes of Africa could be confidently anticipated. In association with scientists from France, Germany, America, Italy and Japan, researchers from Britain made a particularly brilliant contribution to this advance.

Accordingly, I felt a sense of real pride when, as a newly qualified doctor working at the Hospital for Tropical Diseases in London during 1937, I came in contact with such giants in the field as Manson-Bahr, Hamilton Fairley, Carmichael Low, Swinton, Castellani, Scott, Christophers, Wenyon, Chesterman and many others.

It was through the influence of these men, and because the people of Black Africa seemed most in need of help, that I decided to make their continent, and in particular what was then Nyasaland, my field for medical practice. There I very soon learned how terribly disease had sapped and shortened the lives of the lake people and limited their productivity. During foot safaris with my wife, we found one community which exemplified the deplorable infirmity of old Africa. Its people lived in the straggling village of Kachindomoto. The name means 'set the bush on fire', the nom-de-guerre of an old Angoni Chief who nearly a century before had led a pillaging impi from distant Zululand to Lake Nyasa, and there carved out a small principality for himself. We found that every person in Kachindomoto hosted a variety of microscopical animal parasites, and that each man, woman, and child suffered from malnutrition. It was a combination which inevitably drew them into poverty and early graves. To us it seemed that if these conditions were allowed to persist in Africa, its population must perish.

But the very presence of these sickly villagers proclaimed their descent from stock which had been able to maintain itself against these same parasites that had now become their masters. Yet it was some time before I realised that it was the prolonged association between their forbears and local parasites which had led to a selective survival of those more resistant men and women who were protected against the diseases either by chance genetic qualities or by accidental possession of overlapping immunities derived from related infections. Their survival had led to a state of equilibrium between hosts and parasitic clients which allowed them to live together in mutual tolerance, although at the expense of some debility among the Africans. But this situation could only survive so long as the people had little association with strangers.

The equilibrium thus established in Africa was unintentionally destroyed by the European intrusion into the continent. But once the Europeans appreciated the result of their intrusion real efforts were made by the colonial authorities to remedy the position. For it would be wrong to believe that Europe's colonisation of Africa was motivated solely by a desire to exploit the Africans. It became associated too with a growing philanthropic impulse to improve the standard of living of far-away subjects and to lighten their burden of sickness. From the beginning of the present century many men and women went out voluntarily to help Africans, though at the time a posting to Africa must have seemed like a death sentence.

So although Kipling's call to his countrymen and to the Americans to 'Take up the white man's burden' may seem ridiculously quaint and even hypocritical today, there was far more than arrogance and greed in the Powers' attitude to the African people. Indeed it was Kipling himself who best expressed their philanthropic objectives in his most maligned poem, one stanza of which begins:

> Take up the white man's burden,
> The savage wars of peace.
> Fill the mouths of famine
> And bid the sickness cease.

. . . bid the sickness cease. The admonition was heeded by western scientists and they gained considerable success in controlling the infections of Africa, for the period of white

rule of the continent coincided with unparallelled activity
and achievement in the medical field. Pasteur had already
opened up a new world of pathogenic organisms by his
discoveries of 1868, and nine years later Patrick Manson
demonstrated that tropical disease could be transmitted by
biting insects that preyed on man. This was a breakthrough
which gave birth to the new discipline of tropical medicine
and presently allowed the scientists to approach their objective of dispelling the infirmity of Black Africa, a victory
that promised to set its peoples on a new course of prosperity and health. It was no fault of the doctors that in the
end many of the animal parasites of man successfully resisted their attack.

I have here paid special tribute to Manson and his successors who worked so brilliantly, and sometimes at the cost
of their lives, to free the tropics from disease. It is largely
due to their dedication that the African people today have
gained another opportunity to tame their previously hostile
environment and play their part in world affairs, freed at
last from the terrible tyranny of intractable pestilences.

In this book, which greatly relies on original works,
proper reference to them would have required a burden-
some apparatus of footnotes. Instead I have preferred to
provide a list of all the printed sources consulted.

1

Black Africa

THE SHAPE OF AFRICA has always fascinated people: William Blake described the continent as 'heart formed'; others saw its outline as resembling a pear, a simian skull and a fully cocked pistol; the most fanciful of all the commentators likened the profile of the continent to that of an old woman bearing an immense burden on her back, and with her head turned towards the west.

This last impression possesses an aptness denied the others. For the great mass of Africa, that part lying within the tropics, has carried a more grievous burden of disease than any other area in the world, and it very largely determined the history of this vast region.

Africa may be divided into four separate parts. The Mediterranean littoral was once a province of Rome, and its civilisation is drawn from both Christianity and Islam. The southerly tip of Africa is also separate from the mass of the continent; it has long lain under white rule and today South Africa is still part of the western world. A different Africa exists on the high Ethiopian plateau. This region, converted to Christianity during the fourth century, is isolated on two sides by a mountain barrier and an extension of the Sahara desert. Its people possess a high proportion of Caucasian blood and its easy access from the Red Sea led to a life-style influenced by Arabia.

Divided from these three orphaned regions lies the real Africa, Black Africa, that part of the continent which stretches from about 15°N to the Limpopo valley in the south, and it is with this area that we are concerned.

Until the nineteenth century, Black Africa was little more than an outline on maps drawn by speculative cartographers. Admittedly the western seaboard became dotted with the names of commercial entrepôts but they were no more than pestilential toe-holds serving the Atlantic slave trade. On the eastern shores of the continent map-makers also inked in half-mythical names like Sofala, Kilwa, Malindi and Rhapta, which represented ancient Arab ports most of which had long since silted up. But the hinterland of Africa remained a mystery long after China had become known to Europe, and when both America and Australia had been explored. For centuries it remained a blank on the map except for drawings of grotesque animals and cryptic warnings of 'Hic sunt Leones'.

For tropical Africa had lacked the climatic attractions and plunder of the New World, and it proved remarkably difficult to penetrate. There were few deep bays or gulfs along the coast, only scarce headlands to offer shelter to mariners. And most of Africa's rivers were unnavigable because of sand bars at their mouths or rapids a short distance upstream.

Immediately beyond the seaboard, too, lay miles of impassable mangrove swamps, so low lying that a single tree might be the mariner's only landmark for many leagues. Beyond this wilderness of fetid mud grew pathless tropical forests reinforced by thick walls of vegetation. Entrance to the continent was further guarded by savage animals, wilder men and an oppressive climate. Yet by far the most effective factor in keeping Africa inviolate for so long was its diseases. This was recognised during the sixteenth century by a Portuguese archivist who grimly noted that 'it seems for our sins or some inscrutable judgement of God, in all the entrances [into the interior] he has placed a striking angel with a flaming sword of deadly fevers.' These 'deadly fevers' were even more fearsome because the inhabitants of tropical Africa seemed protected against them; their immunity added another psychological barrier to European entry into the interior.

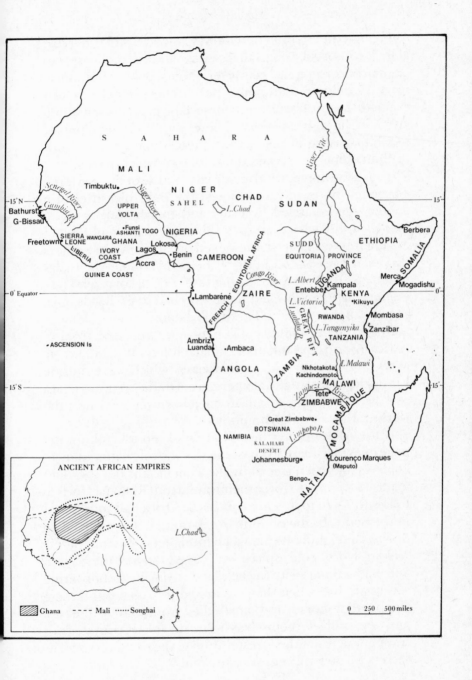

S A H A R A

MALI

Timbuktu.

NIGER   CHAD

SAHEL   L..Chad   SUDAN

15°N
Gambia   15°
Bathurst
G-Bissau   UPPER
                   VOLTA
                   •Funsi   TOGO   NIGERIA
Freetown SIERRA WANGARA ASHANTI   ETHIOPIA
          LEONE   GHANA   Lokosa   Berbera
          IVORY   Accra •Benin   CAMEROON
          COAST Lagos   SUDD
LIBERIA   EQUITORIA PROVINCE
          GUINEA COAST   Merca•
                                                              Mogadishu
0° Equator   •Lambaréné   ZAIRE   L..Albert UGANDA KENYA
                                         Entebbe Kampala
                                         L..Victoria •Kikuyu
                                                RWANDA   Mombasa
                                              L..Tanganyika Zanzibar
          •ASCENSION Is   TANZANIA
                              Ambriz•   ZAMBIA
                              Luanda •Ambaca   Nkhotakota L.Malawi
                                              Kachindomoto•
                              ANGOLA   MALAWI
                                          Tete• ZIMBABWE
15°S   Zambezi River   15°
                              Great Zimbabwe•
                                        BOTSWANA
                              NAMIBIA
                                     KALAHARI
                                     DESERT
                                     Johannesburg•   Lourenço Marques
                                                            (Maputo)
                                         Bengo•
                                              NATAL

Senegal River
Niger River
FRENCH EQUITORIAL AFRICA
Congo River
Luilaba R.
GREAT RIFT
MOÇAMBIQUE
Limpopo R.
River Nile

ANCIENT AFRICAN EMPIRES

L.Chad

▨ Ghana --- Mali ······ Songhai

0   250   500 miles

Though the African hinterland was inaccessible, invisible and incomprehensible there was always great speculation concerning its character. Men spoke of singular marvels hidden there, like the strange bestiary which roamed the continent and whose fabled forms have survived in heraldic devices. There were rumours too of hidden treasure in the African jungles and of the wealth of flourishing native kingdoms, one of which passed into legend as the domain and terrestial paradise of Prester John. There an innocent race enjoyed the pure pleasures of a golden age encircled by cruel and treacherous savages. Medieval wiseacres even spoke about Africa's semi-human inhabitants, some of whom walked on all fours while others had their eyes placed in their chests. No doubt such tales stemmed from Herodotus, the father of history, who had written that men dwelled there who had dogs' heads, presumably a reference to barking baboons.

In fact about eighty million people inhabited tropical Africa towards the end of the nineteenth century but nearly every one was the victim of diseases which were outside European knowledge or experience. For the Africans of last century may be truly said to have been damned into the world rather than born into it.

If the African interior had always been a blank on the page of exploration, its coastline was scarcely better known. Portions had been traced by the Phoenicians but they had made no attempt to force their way inland. Roman efforts to follow the Nile to its source in Black Africa had foundered in the Sudd. In the end the break-in came from the north during the eighth century when foreigners, Moslem traders seeking ivory, gold, spices and slaves, crossed the Sahara and made contact with the black men living in the bordering savannah. But when they attempted to pass beyond these steppes their horses and camels died from strange diseases, and the traders themselves went down with mysterious fevers. As a result the forested land to the south retained its secrets for several centuries to come.*

Co-incident with the Moors' incursion, Indian, Polynes-
ian and Moslem mariners all briefly visited the east African
coast. A few Arab caravans even ventured inland in search
of slaves. Passing fleets of Chinese junks appeared off the
eastern coast at about the same time and bartered exotic
trade goods for rhinoceros horn, ivory and precious stones
which were carried back to China. But contact with the
Africans everywhere was fleeting and casual; the visitors
gained little knowledge of the intrinsic ethos of the interior.
They did not know that beyond the hot, steamy, coastal
plains lay a high, tilted plateau of ancient rock, broken by
several river basins of which the Congo, Zambezi and Niger
are the chief. The plateau is itself bisected by a long geographical fault, the Great Rift Valley. This continuation of
the Jordan Valley and Red Sea extends southward for some
six thousand kilometres, dividing the continent into western
and eastern portions, and determining the eastern boundary
of the tropical rain forest. After broadening in the African
interior to include the spread of the great inland lakes, the
Rift finally debouches into the Indian Ocean near the
mouth of the Zambezi.

To the west of the Great Rift, the African interior is
divided into several regions which merge insensibly into
each other. South of the Sahel, or desert fringe, lies the
northern savannah, a dreary, featureless scrub country
whose stubby grass briefly grows to a man's height during
the rains. These dusty grasslands are dotted with bushes
and trees which can withstand long dry seasons. Scattered
woodlands too appear in the savannah while remnants of

* A notable result of the lack of communication between Black Africa
and its neighbouring continent is the remarkably small number of words
which entered into the European languages. Thus although in English
we think of 'palaver', 'pikinin', and 'fetish' as being of African origin, all
three in fact stem from the Portuguese. Similarly 'kraal' is derived from
the Spanish 'corral', 'chop' is Anglo-Saxon, 'askari' and 'safari' are Arabic,
while 'ju-ju' is the French 'joujou'. Even the word 'compound' is derived
from Malay 'kampong'. 'Dash' and 'mumbo-jumbo' are among the few
introductions that can be accounted authentically African.

ancient forests persist in river valleys. The modern states occupying this area are Mali, Niger, and Chad. Eastwards beyond the rift the savannah curves southwards into what are now Kenya and Tanzania.

The northern savannah gradually changes in the south to the lush, steaming tropical rain forests of west Africa and the Congo basin, extending roughly from 6°N to 6°S. Little sunlight penetrates the canopy of its high trees.

South of the Congo, the forest gives way again to a broad belt of woodland and scrub which stretches across the continent until it becomes debased further south into another wide belt of savannah land that extends beyond the Zambezi valley.

Much of the land in tropical Africa and particularly that in the savannah is of poor quality due to unreliable rainfall and unproductive soil. For centuries the size of the African population in consequence lagged behind that of the smaller continent of Europe. It was only in the forest fringes that settled communities of any size established themselves, while a more nomadic people gained a living from the savannah. Primarily hunters, the nomads also raised cereal crops which were more nutritious than the staples of the forest.

Tsetse flies abounded in the forest, along the rivers and over huge stretches of the savannah, and effectively prevented the rearing of domestic animals. As a result, only human muscle was available for the transportation of goods. The high humidity of the tropical forest and its claustrophobic, sluggish air tended to make its people listless and inclined to a vegetative life, and the warm moist conditions provided breeding grounds for myriads of insects, including those that carried some of the diseases most dangerous to man.

Rainfall varies greatly over Africa. In the coastal plains of the west as many as four hundred inches fall each year, and there is no dry season. A belt of about sixty inches of rain extends to 30° east, and as far south as the Congo River.

Much of the savannah beyond receives an average of thirty inches a year, a figure similar to that of Western Europe, though in Africa the rain is concentrated during the summer months. Vast areas of dry grassland and semi-desert country appear where the rainfall is under twenty inches, and agriculture becomes impossible without irrigation at ten to fifteen inches of rain. Many areas of climatic instability occur in Africa, especially where tree cover has been destroyed. Periods of drought are common there, with resulting malnutrition and increased susceptibility to disease.

Although tropical Africa was long isolated from the main drift of history and progress, it was once the focus of human endeavour and remained a cultural centre until the birth of neolithic civilisation in south-western Asia ten thousand years ago. Evidence suggests that it was in tropical Africa that *homo sapiens* first made his appearance and then spread gradually from Africa into Europe and Asia, learning to keep warm in temperate climates by wearing the skins of other animals as clothing and by domesticating fire. With them at first they carried the parasites of the African forests, but few of these survived in cooler climates which were inimical to them and their vectors. Accordingly the present inhabitants of tropical Africa host a wider variety of human parasites than any other people. In Europe and Asia the emigrants either maintained or acquired a lighter skin.* This allowed them to form sufficient vitamin D to remain healthy despite a low exposure to sunlight. The vitamin is produced in the body by the action of ultra-violet light on its fatty tissues; its deficiency produces rickets.

The people remaining in tropical Africa continued to live in isolation, increasingly cut off from cultural contact with other communities to the north by desiccation of what is

*The members of all human races demonstrate the blush reflex which is associated with courting. This suggests that, following his ancestors' loss of fur, earliest man was pale-skinned. It also indicates that the skin of those who continued to live in the tropics gradually darkened through genetic adaptation in order to prevent the development of harmful amounts of vitamin D which results in hardening of the arteries.

now the Sahara Desert, and the impassability of the upper Nile due to the sudd. Because the members of each group mated with persons possessing similar genes and drew their endowments from a small common pool, they maintained physical characteristics subtly different from those of other races. Yet it is practical to divide the Negroes into two main groups based largely on different language structures. One group comprised the Negroes proper, those people who remained in the tropical forest, and lived by fishing and harvesting root crops, with only a small amount of their energy expended on hunting. The second group consisted of the descendants of the migrants who settled in neighbouring, less constrictive, grasslands. These migrants are now called the Bantu – a philological word coined during the nineteenth century – which comes from *abaNTU* meaning people. The Bantu speak variations of a single root language which differs from that of the forest dwellers.

The Bantu occupy that part of Africa lying roughly below a horizontal line joining the southern limit of the tropical forest to the northern border of Kenya and extending to South Africa. It is believed that the main Bantu migration began from the west coast, skirted both sides of the forest and accelerated when the savannah country was reached in the east. The migrants' expressive language imposed itself on the aboriginal people of the lands they occupied, and was eventually elaborated into four hundred variations, all so similar as to suggest that the Bantu migration was comparatively rapid.

With them the Bantu also carried their infections, and the aborigines they overran, lacking resistance to their diseases, died off. Conquest through the introduction of new diseases to communities lacking any immunity to them became a dominant theme in the unfolding history of tropical Africa.

Three less important people shared Black Africa with the two branches of Negro stock. The most numerous were the light-skinned inhabitants of the Horn of Africa. It is customary still to call these people Hamites; their ancestors are believed to have been of Caucasoid origin and to have originated in the Middle East. Another group – the Capoids or Khoikhoi – comprises the Hottentots and related Bushmen who at one time were spread out through the savannah lands, though their African descendants are today largely confined to the Kalahari desert. Yet another group is made up of the pygmies who still exist in the Congo forests. Some authorities regard these diminutive people as progenitors of the Negro race.

The presence of these five main groups of *homo sapiens* in tropical Africa demonstrates a wider variation of the human form than occurs in Asia or Europe. This polymorphism reflects Africa's comparatively low population density in ancient times which resulted in almost complete lack of contact between the different populations; it prevented the amalgamation of their separate characteristics and for many centuries limited the spread of disease.

The coming of the iron age to Africa equipped the Negroid people with more advanced tools and weapons, and led to a population expansion since cultivation became easier and the earlier trapping of small rodents and the scavenging of carrion for food was replaced by the more profitable hunting of game animals. The iron revolution reached West Africa during the centuries immediately before the Christian era and had spread throughout tropical Africa by the sixth century. Population pressure in the forest lands of western Africa led to the exodus of those people who would become known as the Bantu. These migrants tended to develop somewhat lighter skins and longer legs than their ancestors, possibly because they intermarried with people from the Horn of Africa and because there was a greater emphasis in their lives on running down game in open savannah lands. The absence of tsetse fly in parts of the savannah permitted the raising of cattle, and the Bantu tended to become seasonal farmers in order to exploit the varying climatic conditions.

With singular exceptions the Africans possessed no written languages. All knowledge was stored in the memory and old people, as the custodians of folklore and because of their demonstrable immunity to misfortunes, were highly respected. Their transmission of age-old beliefs by word of mouth led to a remarkable continuity of local cultures.

It is impossible here to do more than generalise over the cultural variations among the main African groups. Common themes may however be identified but every statement is open to qualification, and nearly all of them should be followed by the words 'with notable exceptions'.

Generally the Africans were communalists whose first affiliation was to the family, then to clan and finally to the group or tribe. But some of the Negroes in the northern savannah, who were exposed to periodic nomadic incursions across the Sahara, found safety by living in larger communities, akin to European states.

From Arab travellers' accounts we know a good deal about these black 'empires' in the bulge of Africa below the desert fringe, which all exhibited a similar pattern of expansion and decline. The empire of Ghana was one of the first to appear and reached its peak of power about AD 1000. It lay between the Senegal River and the upper Niger, many hundreds of miles north-west of modern Ghana. Ghana's power was based on the control of the route along which the gold mined at Wangara in the south was carried to the Sahara and then on to Morocco.

Ghana's decline was followed by the rise of the empire of Mali, whose African rulers became converted to Islam. One of them, Mansa Musa, made a well-publicised pilgrimage to Mecca during 1325. His second city was Timbuktu, then a centre of African trade and learning. Mali was succeeded by the Songhai empire which at one time stretched from the mouth of the Gambia River almost to Lake Chad. Songhai was conquered by Moroccan troops in 1589 and its fall signalled the end of the powerful states of the sahel, though less formidable confederations appeared later during the middle of last century round Lake Chad and in the northern parts of modern Ghana.

From Arab reports we gain the impression that the medieval states of the sahel were prosperous and well governed. Unfortunately we know very little about the nature and prevalence of disease among them, but because few of the inhabitants lived in the pestilential forest, and those in the comparatively healthy sahel adopted the clothes and hygienic habits of their Moslem rulers, they probably suffered no more severely from disease than contemporary Europeans.

The formation of centralised states was less common among the Bantu, although there were notable exceptions like the empire of Monomatapa in modern Zimbabwe. This state reached its pinnacle of power in about 1450, while its successor states remained viable until the beginning of the nineteenth century. Portuguese travellers' accounts suggest that its people were robust and virile and did not suffer unduly from disease.

Before the European conquest in the late nineteenth century, however, the great majority of Africans were stateless. They were held together in a multitude of small communities by virtue of relationship, close proximity, kinship, neighbourhood arrangements and village circumstances. These components were the dynamics of African life and more important than any feeling of national or even tribal identity. The fragmentary character of the population's distribution and ethos is reflected today by the twenty ethnic groups living in the modern state of Guinea-Bissau, all of which have differences in their social structures, beliefs and cultural values.

There existed well over seven hundred tribal groupings in Africa, all of them significantly different in culture, size and power. Each had its own means of raising food, of dealing with disputes, even of interring the dead. Each spoke a separate language and this diversity of tongues denied the African another important unifying force. Villagers living within a few kilometres of each other might be unable to communicate, and it was inevitable that when Europeans entered the continent, few found it expedient to learn any of the innumerable languages they encountered until the missionaries undertook the study of linguistics so that they might preach the Gospel. In eastern Africa, however, a *lingua franca*, ki-swahili, which included many Arabic loan words, did develop; on the west coast, foreigners found they could best get along with pidgin English.

Another important characteristic must be recognised in African life. Groups of people were held together as much by kinship with the dead as with the living. By 1890 some converts had been made by Islam and Christianity, but the majority of Africans, while acknowledging the existence of a Supreme Being, still worshipped their remote and immediate tribal ancestors, as well as inanimate objects and natural phenomena; in addition the people had their own naiads and dryads, spirits inhabiting lakes, mountains and forests. They had faith in prolonging earthly life through procreation. They looked upon their bodies as little more than garments which sheltered their spirits that were immortal. Individuals believed that death provided a new and superior position which could be used to defend their homes, allow them to take part in the affairs of the living and mete out punishment to their descendants when required.

The ratio of men to women in Black Africa towards the end of the last century was ninety-five to a hundred, which differed significantly from that of other races. (In India, for instance, the ratio is one hundred and three males to each hundred females.) Perhaps this factor was due to African women being more resilient than the men and living longer. In 1890 the population was predominantly rural. The Africans lived rhythmical, low-tempo lives which had not changed for centuries. As elsewhere in the world, the great mass of peasants was gripped in the vice of poverty. Life was controlled by their hungers, their desires, and the need to protect their crops and persons. They enjoyed little privacy; eating, sleeping, cooking, working, sometimes even making love, were conducted in public. Most were subsistence farmers, subject always to the down-drag of leached soil, unreliable rains and mystifying agricultural diseases. Their crops were constantly at risk too, from pests which ranged from packs of baboons to swarms of locusts. The spectre of famine hung always over them. Life balanced on a razor edge of chance.

The Africans, being settled in small self-subsistence communities made up of one or more family units, avoided inbreeding by forbidding marriage between members of the same kin or totem. Incest was in some cases punishable by death. The men were polygamous which was necessary for group survival when child mortality was high. Polygamy also avoided a surplus of women but it jeopardized the advantageous results of natural selection. Thus a person who was mentally backward or possessed poor physical genes, would nevertheless be likely to mate and propagate undesirable traits. On the other hand the Africans were essentially conformist, diligently avoiding emphasis and inclined to be antagonistic to obvious deviates like albinos. This may have accounted for the absence among Africans of cleft palates and pelvic bony abnormalities through lessening of gene diversity, although the potentially advantageous possession of additional fingers still occurs among small groups of people in Africa.

The conformance to tradition arose from a pervading fear of the spirits who were believed to frown on innovation: their unceasing influence bred mental discipline, fortitude, and self-denial, as well as lack of initiative or ambition. On the credit side it resulted in the Africans developing a strong sense of community. Of necessity so much of their time was spent in acquiring food or propitiating the ancestral spirits that little was left for intellectual pursuits. Few questions were asked, few doubts raised, and curiosity was discouraged by the tribal elders lest it challenged their authority. And so, because the inhabitants of Old Africa sustained a culture of acceptance and encountered the minimum of novel experiences, the already conservative pressures of society tended to be perpetuated and made them highly resistant to change.

The African women were prolific, falling pregnant at an early age and bearing large numbers of children. Tragically, many of these would die during infancy. By the age of thirty most women were worn out by continuous childbearing. Even in widowhood they became the property of their dead husband's nearest male relative and might bear more offspring. The women's duties were heavy; beside tending the local staple crop, they also accepted the chores of pounding grain, tending subsidiary crops, hewing wood, drawing water, making pots and searching the bush for edible relishes. The men concerned themselves with hunting, herding or fishing, building huts or canoes, and sometimes with fighting.

Human mortality was as brutally high as in India and other undeveloped tropical regions. Not many Africans lived beyond the age of forty*; grey heads were rarely seen. Even in 1890 the peasants possessed few material goods. Many went unshod; some were naked; the more fortunate were clad in animal skins, or bark 'cloth' which was made from figtrees and beautifully worked. But again there were exceptions: the Yoruba for instance were turning out excellent cotton cloth by the sixteenth century. Currency hardly existed except for rare objects like cowrie shells derived from the Maldives. Hoes were, however, a medium of exchange among the agricultural Bantu, although perhaps not strictly as currency since they were insufficiently

---

* Nor did they in England three thousand years ago. Of thirty-five skeletons excavated at Maiden Castle, eleven were those of infants, nineteen under the age of forty, four between forty and forty-five, and only one over forty-five.

abstract. (An Austrian mission, which benevolently introduced a million hoes into southern Mozambique, destroyed
at a stroke the whole social fabric of marriage payments.) In
an iron-using system, bars of iron functioned similarly as
money, in the same way as silver did elsewhere in the world
until the ultimate abstraction of paper money appeared.
Bartering was common and among the Bantu, cattle were
looked on as a form of wealth or, perhaps more correctly,
regarded as westerners cherish jewellery.

Most Africans live in simple, round huts, usually of mud
with thatched roofs. These were windowless, lacked effective
illumination at night and were smoky from the slow fires
maintained in the centre of the limited living space. They
lived in close contact with the earth; it was their chair, their
bed, their table. Manufactured domestic furniture was
minimal, agricultural tools crude. Individual holding of
ground did not exist in most societies. The people had not
learned the technology of harnessing the wind to crush
grain or run a mill; all tasks depended on human muscle.
There was rarely any social status other than village senior-
ity and cattle wealth, though many Bantu paid some alleg-
iance to a distant chief. Yet everywhere African life was
graced by great dignity, inherent delicacy of feeling, and
traditional wisdom. In some areas culture was highly advanced, as is demonstrated by the Benin bronzes, Ashanti
gold weights and the brass figures from Dahomey.

Social life was subtle and highly complex. Alcohol played
an important part in the communal round. Beer, sometimes
so thick as to resemble gruel, assisted in the fulfilment of
religious and social functions, as well as in the organisation
of collective work. Liquor was also used as payment for
labour of medical treatment and as a means of sacrificing to
the family ancestors; no less important, it provided a valuable source of vitamins B and C. African recreations were
limited, but they particularly enjoyed their music and
dancing, sometimes in an attempt to gain communication
with their ancestors but more often for the sheer basic

pleasure it gave them to keep in time with the insistent beaten rhythm of the village drums.

The growth of agriculture during the iron age, first in the forests and then in the savannah, required the African families to live in small groups near their holdings, which they usually called 'gardens'. Land, being communal, was allotted to each family according to its need. Droughts were frequent, and these were often accompanied by disastrous invasions of locusts. Farming methods were crude and inefficient. Crop rotation was not practised. Fertilisation was limited to the use of night soil, the rare manure and routine bush burning which provided only temporary reinforcement of minerals in the soil. The Africans' domesticated animals comprised goats, donkeys, guinea-fowl and chickens as well as those breeds of cattle which were immune to tsetse-fly disease. They possessed only crude facilities for storing surplus crops, and these provided little protection against rodents and insects. Accordingly, the inclination was to plant only sufficient seed for immediate needs. Compared with its frequent use in Asia and Egypt, irrigation was little practised except in parts of East Africa.

In very early times the Africans cultivated the indigenous yams and gourds, and probably millet and sorghum. Sugar cane reached the continent from Asia at about the same time as the banana, of which over twenty varieties are grown in Uganda, suggesting that it has been cultivated there for at least two thousand years. Rice was introduced from Asia during the seventh century. New food crops from the Americas began entering tropical Africa soon after the discovery of the New World; of these maize was by far the most important and its cultivation spread rapidly through Black Africa; other imports from America included sweet potatoes, paw paws, ground nuts, and cassava (manioc). Cassava possesses an important advantage: it is easily preserved and carried as 'journey food'. This allowed long expeditions and migrations to be undertaken, and thus it became a factor in the spread of disease. However it has been suggested by some people that it possesses one particular disadvantage: if taken in large quantities it affects the secretion of the thyroid gland.

Fruits were generally rare, but there was a great reliance on nuts, wild roots and plants which were added to a meal as relish. First-class protein was mainly obtained from eating termites, grasshoppers and other insects, and by recourse to snails, caterpillars and lizards.

The staples only provided the African with the required daily number of calories if consumed in large quantities. Unfortunately this was seldom possible during the hungry months preceding the harvest. Moreover, the staples were deficient in protein, iron, calcium, amino-acids and B-complex vitamins. As a result most of the Africans suffered to some extent from malnutrition, this being especially manifest among children whose bodily growth depended largely on a good supply of nutritive factors.

Although suffering from some degree of vitamin shortage, the children were most seriously affected by protein-calorie deficiency. This caused a condition which scientists called kwashiorkor. It is a Ghanaan word meaning 'disease which the young child developed when displaced from his mother by another child or pregnancy'. The condition is characterised by general swelling of the body and protusion of the belly, together with sparseness and reddish colouring of the hair.

Kwashiorkor most generally affected infants weaned from the breast and not yet able to cope with an adult diet. It still occurs throughout the tropics in developing countries. Thus a recent survey showed an incidence of seven per cent in Haiti, and probably a similar figure occurred in precontact Africa, though it must to some extent have been avoided by the women's prolonged lactation and the proscription of intercourse until the latest baby was weaned. Kwashiorkor greatly lessens a child's resistance to infection.

These people of Old Africa had, for centuries, lived their lives at subsistence level, and although generally free from the 'crowd diseases' of large population concentrations, they were continually exposed to virulent tropical infections, most of which were transmitted by some vector such as mosquito, tsetse fly or snail. Fortunately, over many generations, the people had acquired a considerable degree of immunity to these diseases, and many survived them, although at the expense of some debility and mortality. To unfamiliar and old infections in previously inaccessible areas, however, they were highly vulnerable, and against them they possessed no preventive or therapeutic measures of any value. After Africa was 'opened up' by Europe, its peoples frequently encountered such new disease-bearing organisms. These took a terrible human toll as was very evident to me on my arrival in the Continent.

I shall never forget my first encounter with the poverty and infirmity of Africa. That introduction took place shortly before the outbreak of the Second World War. My wife and I were stationed at the time on the rim of the high plateau which overlooks Lake Malawi from the west, and my duties as a government medical officer took me frequently to the 'rural dispensaries' scattered along the lakeshore. During my first 'ulendo' (journey of inspection) I arrived at the dusty village of Kachindomoto at the head of an imposing line of porters whose headloads included a field-kitchen, tent, bed, bath, clothes and food. As I made my way towards the small brick building which served as a dispensary I found myself followed by a shuffling throng of sick people, who, I was to find, were stoically resigned to a lifetime of sickness and poverty.

Emaciated children stood among the growing crowd on legs so thin and fragile as to resemble dry twigs, hardly capable, it seemed, of supporting the bloated bellies now so familiar to us, by television exposure, as the plight of refugees all over the world. These children had just eaten their morning meal which consisted only of left-overs from their parents' supper of the night before. It was no wonder that they suffered from malnutrition. Beside them, steadying frail bodies with staffs like medieval pilgrims, stood taller human spectres who were mutely peeling off dirty rags to expose tropical ulcers which were eating away their legs. Other men and women came hobbling up on feet half destroyed by jigger fleas. A score of people were suffering from dripping eye infections. Others exhibited deformities like figures out of a Hieronymus Bosch painting.

The scene this day at Kachindomoto was to remain imprinted on my memory with that peculiar intensity of inner vision which allows it to be recalled instantly and without effort. It was a microcosm of conditions in the heartland of Africa, and it came to us as a painful shock. To deepen our concern we learned that these forgotten people of the world, who were almost all suffering from multiple infections, were well aware that waves of killer diseases like measles and meningitis might also strike their village at any time with terrible results. Sometimes as I recall that village crowd, I think gratefully that within thirty years new remedies and preventive measures against disease would' have begun to transform the quality of life in Africa. As it was, once we had recovered from our distress, my wife and I dressed the patients' wounds, gave injections to a lucky few from the magical syringe which they held in such high regard, and handed out draughts of medicine and little packets of pills. Then I was led to a nearby hut infested, as I would learn later, with the organisms responsible for several tropical diseases; in it a woman lay groaning in complicated labour far beyond the power of the village midwife to correct. Nearby in another hut sprawled a child so near to death from dysentery that only her sunken eyes seemed alive, and at a third I peered through the pungent gloom to where a man lay wasting away from a fly-blown wound. As the morning wore on it seemed that every other hut in the village sheltered an invalid.

That afternoon, having inspected the local lunatics who were restrained from violence by being chained to heavy logs so they could only move with difficulty, we watched the barefooted 'healthy' workers come padding back to the village from distant gardens, and winced again to see that their skin was so dry and cracked as to resemble a variegated mosaic – another clear sign of chronic malnutrition. Behind them came a line of trance-like women gliding along with laden pots and 'debbies' (old petrol cans) on their heads. They were returning from the local water point which turned out to be heavily infected with bilharzia. Later I would learn that every single villager suffered from this, the great dibilitating disease of Africa, and parents thought it normal for their children to pass blood in their urine. I would also discover that these village women spent thirteen per cent of their time obtaining water for their families.

All the men were of small stature, a head shorter than Europeans of the same age, stunted by the poor food available to them during childhood and weakened by near starvation during the vital planting seasons. As Dr B.S. Platt reported in a nutritional survey in a nearby village that same year, 'at a time when food stocks were low and the energy expended in operations at the opening of an agricultural season was high, the energy value of the food eaten was only sixty per cent of the estimated requirement'.

When, at the outbreak of the Second World War, recruiting for the King's African Rifles began on the lakeshore almost all the men seen were suffering from multiple infections and only a few were considered fit for service, though army rations soon improved their condition considerably.

But had we come to Kachindomoto eighty years earlier we would have witnessed a very different scene. The village would then have been thronged with strutting Angoni warriors carrying huge ox-hide shields and the stabbing assegais of Zululand. The air would have been loud with the beat of war drums and shouted praise songs for their induna. These men had been of splendid physique, the black skins shining with health. They were noted for their endurance, each one capable of covering fifty miles on foot every day for a week on end.

The warriors had been evicted from their home in Natal by Chaka Zulu during 1819. They had then marched like vengeful furies through Central Africa disrupting successive communities, even pillaging Great Zimbabwe itself. They looted without mercy and killed everyone who crossed their paths, except for nubile girls and youths considered fit to recruit into their growing impis. By 1834 the Angoni had reached Lake Tanganyika, and there one section turned back to settle on the shores of Lake Malawi, where one of the indunas, Kachindomoto, set up his own small fief centred on the village where my dispensary would later stand. From this stronghold his impi every year would storm through the district to 'set the bush on fire', mercilessly raiding for crops, cattle and women. But when we came to Kachindomoto in 1938 these exciting forays had long since ceased; the old vitality of the Angoni had been slowly drained from them by disease against which they possessed no immunity. It seemed ironical to us that these warriors of a century before, had become victims of village parasites which they could not even see – the revenge perhaps of the lakeshore people they had displaced.

The scene around the dispensary was very different too from the image of Africa I had conjured up after reading of the stable states of the interior which had been so vividly described by early Arab and European explorers. They had stressed the civil order they found in domains like Mali and Monomatapa. Travellers wrote then of the 'respectable and opulent' cities they had seen and of the 'elegance and state' of rulers like the successive Casembes and the priestly kings of great Zimbabwe. These potentates had controlled considerable armies, and the physique and vitality of their soldiers had greatly impressed their visitors. All that, it seemed, had changed. I remembered too on our first visit to Kachindomoto that the Portuguese nobles treated the kings of Mani-Kongo as equals and allies. I recalled that the

Ashanti developed a land code whose sophistication approached that of the Norman conquerors in England, and that the ruling dynasty of Buganda extended over twenty generations. Throughout Africa, up to Livingstone's time, white visitors apart from slavers had treated its people with respect, though only fifty years later they would regard the 'natives' as 'naturally inferior'. I recollected that Quelimane was once a town of 'haughty gentlemen', Benin a city so large that it was traversed by a road fully five kilometres long, while Kano, according to Hugh Clapperton, 'may contain thirty thousand to forty thousand residents'. The people of such states had been cohesive, confident, xenophobic, and vigorously artistic. As I stood in Kachindomoto, I conjured up the names of the other old empires of Africa: they sounded like distant drum beats – Adansi, Dahomey, Oyo, Akan, Guruhuswa and Denkyira, all of them now vanished.

Clearly then, something dreadful had happened to rural Africa during the past sixty years, and I would have to discover what it was. These people I watched with such distress in that lakeshore village had scarcely known a single day's health during their lives. They had not offended anyone; they were not malefactors; they were simply persons who had been born in Africa when the toll of sickness had become extremely high. And yet they bore their burden of disease with remarkable stoicism. To them it was part of another worldly plan against which it was useless to struggle. Over and over again in eastern Africa I would hear an African when overcome by some disaster explain it unemotionally as *Shauri la Mungu* – it is God's will and His responsibility. Their helpless acceptance of misfortune and disease struck me as standing in poignant contrast to the African's natural gaiety and easily aroused enthusiasm.

Shauri la Mungu was a statement about the awesome inevitability of disaster during life, an expression which bears some relation to the *moira* of the Greeks, the *fatum* of Rome and the *kismet* of Islam. The Shona have a similar expression, *mdi Midzimu* (it is the gods), and the Venda intone *zwi di itwa* (that is what has been done).

The Africans' mental surrender to inexorable fate struck me as being very different from the sub-conscious (yet cherished) belief held by many Europeans I knew that they were the pivotal centre of the universe. This central illusion, the logically indefensible fantasy of being the focal point of the cosmos, was for them a vital possession, for without it these white men would be lost. Perhaps because the African considered himself to be less individualistic than Europeans, but rather a part of a greater whole, he did not require the central illusion for survival.

If their poor physical condition seemed hardly their concern, I asked as I pressed them further, but rather a case of *Shauri la Mungu*, did they then worship a god? It was only sometime later after several years soldiering with African units that I came to understand that they did indeed believe in a single deity that had created the world, but had subsequently relinquished responsibility for its salvation. The globe and all that lived thereon had instead been handed over to the care of supernatural forces. These spirits were themselves created parts of the living world, and each one of them was concerned with particular commitments.

It seemed to me that those Africans I questioned regarded their lives as but a prelude to a presumably more rewarding spiritual life, although for the time being they were surrounded by a multitude of mysterious dangers. The concept allowed them to rationalise the poverty and huge toll of disease from which they suffered. They would not admit that illness resulted from natural causes; instead it was the result of the intrusion of magical forces, often instigated by human enemies and manipulated by members of the spirit world, from which their ancestral spirits were sometimes able, though not always inclined, to protect them. These stricken people rarely asked what had caused an illness but rather who induced it – a neighbour with a grudge, a witch, a spirit. It was a concept which through the ages had held people back from seeking a rational explanation for the illnesses that beset them.

Lacking any scientific insight into the causes of diseases, the Africans I spoke to seemed to have remained at the same state of therapeutic knowledge as my own medieval ancestors who also believed implicitly in witchcraft as the cause of any illness.

It must be remembered in the context of this African attitude to illness that only a few centuries ago witches were burnt at the stake in Europe and the king's touch was generally believed to cure scrofula (though not necessarily by the chief participant, for William III when performing the ceremony was heard to mutter 'God grant them better health and more sense.') Church bells were rung in Britain during epidemics, not for religious reasons, but to disperse the polluted air. Amulets were long popular in old England: her people carried a foot of a mole in their pockets to ward off cramp and a potato to prevent rheumatism, while a bag of peonies hung round the neck could be relied on to propitiate evil spirits. In Europe church ceremonies were commonly held for casting out the demons which caused illness, while saintly patrons for most diseases were recognised, and their supernatural intervention solicited in all illnesses and misfortunes. Thus prayers were offered to the martyred St Laurence by sufferers from lumbago, since, while being roasted on a spit, the saint asked to be turned over because his back was well cooked. The intervention of St Sebastion was regularly invoked during visitations of the plague, because he had been slain by arrows which in the Middle Ages were represented as the conveyors of disease. St Lazarus, that 'certain beggar . . . full of sores', whom Jesus healed of leprosy was venerated as its saint; his name lingers on at St Lazarre in Paris and the Venetian island of San Lazarro. Victims of toothache invoked help from St Apollonia whose teeth had been knocked out by a rioting mob. There were many other examples of medieval saintly patrons of disease, the most engaging of whom was perhaps St Fiacre who guarded against piles and unaccountably gave his name to a type of Paris taxi-cab.

Even today rheumatic sufferers wear copper bangles on their wrists and proclaim their efficacy, while suspicious people will grope around to touch wood after boasting unwisely of their good health. In practice some old fashioned remedies in Europe turned out to be surprisingly effective; thus foxglove tea, which contained digitalis, was advantageously prescribed for dropsy, and it was good practice to use cow dung to poultice whitlows. Unfortunately, however, until quite recently in Europe 'brisk' bleeding was the universal remedy for most complaints, although it can only have harmed and often finished off the unhappy patient.

So although the Africans' ideas about disease were not very different from those of our own European ancestors, they had developed them along subtly different lines. Those of them I questioned appeared to recognise four kinds of illness and disability. The first group consisted of uncomplicated wounds and fractures which they regarded as affecting only the physical man; these mishaps could be treated by ordinary members of the community using simple remedies like bandaging and splinting. Then there were some conditions due to injury of the person's life spirit, and these were believed to be best treated by herbal remedies. Thirdly, some people suffered from disease following injury to the breath spirit while a fourth group's diseases resulted from damage to the intrinsic human soul.

Illnesses of these last two groups followed disrespect shown either to the patient's ancestral guardians or tribal spirits, and they were best treated with arcane ceremonies which were accompanied by music and dancing, or by making sacrifices at their forebears' graves.

Such rituals often entailed assistance from the spirit mediums or traditional healers in the community. The mediums were holy men of a kind, highly important and

respected figures of the local establishment, and however
sceptical one may be at first, an observer of their powers
could not fail to be impressed. I have watched these healers
fall into a trance at a meeting with a sick man and his
relatives. During it the medium communicated with the
spirit of the disease, or with an ancestral spirit. Then to the
accompaniment of singing, dancing and prayer, the advice
and wishes of the spirit would be communicated to the
congregation and presently the patient would pronounce
himself cured.

The magic men were known by numerous names
throughout sub-Saharan Africa: in the eastern savannah it
was usually a derivative of the root *nganga*. (*Nganga* means a
cow horn, in which the doctors carried their medicaments.)
European visitors often spoke slightingly of them as 'witch
doctors', and indeed they sometimes did proclaim their
profession in a bizarre fashion, often with a heap of strange
dried objects set up higgledy-piggledy before them on the
ground – a jackal's jawbone, a tiny pile of monkey's teeth
or a dissicated tortoise head. The diviners were profound
psychologists. Many threw bones to discover the cause of
their clients' maladies or to discover the nature of their
errors, while sagely assessing the patient's emotions and
reactions. In times of drought these men also presided over
rain-making ceremonies.

For a fee the medicine men would provide amulets or
fetishes to protect their clients against disease or misfortune. These often took the form of a small, square skin
pouch containing animal remains and generally darkened
by age. They were worn on the body, usually round the arm,
wrist or neck.

These practitioners also purveyed a battery of charms;
some of them would ensure success in the chase or court-
ship; there were others to contrive victory in battle or injure
an enemy. The names given to these talismans varied
throughout Africa; on the west coast they were known as
gris-gris and *juju*. They might be anything from a dried

mouse impaled on a stick to a raffia doll, or a nailparing from the intended victim.

It has been noticed that injury to the life spirit, the inate dignity and aura of a person, required consultation with doctors who specialised in dispensing herbal remedies gathered under prescribed conditions, including the murmuring of secret incantations. Their nostrums were concoctions of tree barks, plant roots, stems, bulbs, fruits and flowers to which might be added pulverised animal parts. They were presented to the patient by mouth, in local application after skin scarification, by inhalation, or as enemas.

Malaria, a common complaint, was treated seemingly effectively by the herbalists of some areas with infusions made from the bark of the croton tree. Elsewhere therapeutic sweating was induced by placing the blanketed patient over a steaming vapour bath containing herbs, cardamon and pepper. Dr Livingstone was once subjected to this vapour treatment but ruefully decided that quinine therapy was far superior.

The African herbalists possessed a wide-ranging pharmacopoeia. They treated rheumatism by local scarification of the skin into which powdered balms and capsicum were rubbed; it was a logical way of providing counter-irritation. Several herbal remedies were effective for dysentery. In ear infections the juice from the plant commonly called mother-in-law's tongue was instilled into the affected ear. Purging enemas, administered through a cow horn (or in the case of infants a reed) were in common use for undiagnosed maladies. Excessive or painful menstruation was alleviated by an infusion of wild gladioli leaves; toothache responded to a paste made from *Wadelia natalensis*; bleeding was prescribed for headaches, and tincture of Buchu for urinary complaints. A form of vaccination against smallpox was practised in some regions, while in West Africa the pustules were smeared with palm oil and isolation practised. Powdered leaves of *Datura stramonium* in solution was beneficially prescribed for asthma. Filariasis was treated with an infusion of catchthorn (*Ziziphus abyssinica*) which doubled as an abortifacient. The unripe fruit of the surrealistic sausage tree (*Kigelia pinnata*) was used for both syphilis and rheumatism, while failing eyesight was said to respond to an infusion of *Bauhinia macrantha* and herpes to local applications made from the bark of *Balanitis aegyptica*. So effective were some of these prescriptions that the same ones came into general use throughout large areas of Africa.

The folk doctors were psychologists as persuasive as any snake-oil vendors and well fitted to relieve neurotic conditions. Many were deft with their hands. Functional tourniquets were applied for snake bites, complicated fractures were carefully splinted, and open wounds sewn up with a series of short thorn barbs. The doctors were particularly skilful at removing jigger fleas from septic toes, and at lassoing the heads of guinea worms as they emerged from a leg, followed by slow winding of the worms around sticks for days on end until they were completely extracted.

Despite their ignorance of anatomy, in some areas local surgeons displayed remarkable skills. The Masai of Kenya for instance showed great facility in performing amputations.

In the Congo, Sir Roger Casement was interested to watch the dexterity with which 'medicine men' removed the enlarged glands that occur in sleeping sickness: 'after feeling the hard lumps embedded in the muscle round the back of the neck and in the glands of the throat,' he wrote, they 'worked them up clear of the veins and then with a rough country-made lancet opened them up to view.' Then Casement continued, 'a needle was used to pass a thread through each lump, by which it was withdrawn.' The use of alcohol as an anaesthetic was well known, and bleeding from a wound was effectively controlled by the application of melted butter or red-hot stones, and occasionally by the use of compresses made from cobwebs. Even caesarian sections were performed in Uganda. A medical student named

Felkin who was in the country during 1879 watched a successful section completed so smoothly by an operating team that it could only have resulted from long practice.

Felkin left us an account describing their methods, of how the patient's abdomen was first washed with banana wine before a deep incision was made straight through the skin and uterine wall. This manoeuvre was accompanied by a shrill cry from all those gathered outside the village 'operating theatre', a demonstration that appeared to be an integral part of the operation.

Bleeding was then dealt with by the application of hot irons before the child was extracted. Manual compression of the uterus was next applied but the organ was not sewn up because, it was explained, of the risk from sepsis. The skin wound was closed by the insertion of a series of small polished iron 'spikes', after which the area was covered with root paste before being tightly bandaged. The spikes were removed in two sessions on the third and fifth post-operative days and the patient thereafter made a rapid recovery.

Yet for all their skills the Africans had no specific remedies for the killer infections to which they were exposed, and they were incapable of remedying the malnutrition from which so many of them suffered. They could not organise themselves to fight or prevent disease, for although African culture did instil a duty towards sick relatives, there was little obligation to help strangers who fell ill. Moreover, among many communities, attendance on invalids was repugnant since it entailed soiling the hands with which they took their food.

At the time of our first visit to the lakeshore in Malawi we were well aware that the battle against disease in Africa had already begun and that it had become scientifically directed. But we did not realise that even greater therapeutic advances lay only a few years in the future, and that when we left Kachindomoto that evening, tropical Africa stood poised on a threshold of medical discovery which would promise to lift from it the immense burden of infirmity.

2

The Infirmity of Africa

SOON AFTER OUR ARRIVAL in Africa the demands of the
Second World War carried me from one end of the continent to the other, and a growing familiarity with Africa's
infirmity led me to attempt a categorisation of those diseases
which caused so much suffering. Eventually I committed
them to five different classes.

The first comprised those illnesses which were either fatal
or affected their victims semi-permanently and so prevented them from earning a living. It was these infections
which were a prime factor in preventing Africa's due
development. They consisted of malaria, sleeping sickness
(trypanosomiasis), bilharzia (schistosomiasis), hook worm
infestation (ankylostomiasis), filariasis and river blindness
(onchocerciasis).

The next most important group included those diseases
whose lesser severity allowed their victims to support themselves, yet so lowered their vitality as to reduce their work
output and expectation of life. These were the two forms of
dysentery (amoebic and bacillary), various forms of skin
ulceration (those caused by jigger fleas and the mysterious
tropical ulcers were the most debilitating and widespread),
worm infestations other than ankylostomiasis, yaws and
leprosy.

These two groups of disease exerted an important
secondary effect. By diminishing the energy potential of the
individual African they adversely affected crop production.
This led to reduced intake of calories, followed by general
apathy and malnutrition, especially among growing children who require comparatively large amounts of vitamins
for normal development. Accordingly malnutrition can be

regarded as the most common medical condition in Black Africa, and one which made the people prone to non-tropical infections of which pneumonia, bronchitis and tuberculosis would prove the most dangerous.

The third group comprised the epidemic scourges of Africa which appear when certain biological and environmental factors are favourable. This list included typhus, plague, yellow fever, smallpox, relapsing fever, and cerebro-spinal meningitis.

The fourth group was made up of those diseases that have been introduced into rural Africa from outside, such as cholera, syphilis and gonorrhoea. To these conditions the Africans possessed no built-in resistance.

The final group comprised other introduced maladies which are particularly common in the western world. They affected tropical Africa especially after industrialisation herded whole sectors of the population into close contact. Among this class were influenza, measles and pneumonia.

It may be noted in parenthesis that the African disease pattern differed from that of Europeans outside the context of tropical illnesses, though it is perhaps related to different environmental conditions. Thus we found that the rural African rarely suffered from stomach ulcers, hardening of the arteries, varicose veins, piles, gall-bladder disease, raised blood pressure, enlargement of the prostate gland, and cancer of the stomach or intestines, all of them common for example among Europeans and Americans. It must be accepted that to some extent the differing incidence arose from the Africans' shorter life-span.

On the other hand Africans are especially prone to cirrhosis of the liver, cancer of the oesophagus or liver, Burkitt's tumour (a recently discovered growth affecting the lymph glands of African children) and a group of cardiac diseases characterised by fibrosis of the heart muscle, the latter it is believed due to a reactive process to malaria.

But it is with tropical diseases that this book is mainly concerned, and what seemed most striking about the

categories into which I had arranged them was the realisation that the first two groups, which included the most
virulent of the African infections, were nearly all caused by
small animal parasites. Some of these are large enough to be
seen by the naked eye, others like the malaria parasite in its
earliest stage are measured in microns (millionths of a
metre), and are only revealed by a microscope's high-power
lens. Of the remaining illnesses mentioned, most are due to
bacteria (which are also measured in microns), but three of
them, including yellow fever, are caused by viruses which are
so small that they are measured in thousandths of a micron.

The appreciation that tiny animal parasites are responsible for the most serious diseases affecting the Africans led
to our seeking a working definition of both animals and
animal parasites together with an appreciation of their
differences from plants.

From a dictionary, I learned that an animal is a living
organism endowed with sensation and free movement. It
derives its food from plants and from other animals. Its
metabolic processes depend on the absorption of oxygen
and the giving off of carbon dioxide. Besides being motile,
an animal usually alters its shape under stimulation.

Plants differ from animals in generally being devoid of
locomotary powers, special organs of sensation, and of a
digestive tract. They manufacture their food by photo-
synthesis, turning carbon dioxide into oxygen. The bacteria
which cause many of the metropolitan diseases are plants.

Unhappily, further consideration showed that these
definitions were too facile. Some of the disease organisms
show no clear-cut distinction between plant and animal.
Thus the spirochaetes (bacteria which are spiral-shaped)
are scientifically plants but yet enjoy free movement and in
this respect resemble animals. In fact scientists now regard
the most important distinction between the plant and
animal worlds as the tougher cell walls of plants which are
more rigid than those of animals due to their higher content
of cellulose.

Viruses are another type of living, disease-bearing, organism, and to complicate matters further, they cannot be regarded as either plant or animal. Their remote ancestors were mere molecules of nucleic acid and protein. Viruses are the smallest of all living organisms, able to pass through porcelain or asbestos filters which would block the passage of bacteria. They are too minute to be seen through an ordinary microscope, but are revealed by electron-microscopy. Among the diseases caused by viruses are poliomyelitis, influenza, shingles, mumps and chicken-pox. A virus infection may confer life-long immunity to its disease. In order to survive and reproduce itself, most viruses therefore require rapid transfer from one human host to another; accordingly many virus diseases did not become serious menaces to tropical Africa because most of its communities, a century ago, were too small to support viral infections. It was only after the African population increased and there was more contact with outsiders that these infections became common in the continent.

It must be repeated that what was most notable about my classification of diseases was that all those listed in the first group were due to animal parasites. Of the second group, amoebic dysentery and worm infections were also caused by animal parasites; bacteria were responsible for bacillary dysentery and leprosy, while yaws is caused by spirochaetes which balance on the border line between plant and animal life.

One must pause here briefly again to consider the phenomenon of parasitism which is important to the proper understanding of disease, particularly in tropical Africa. Terrestial life is maintained by an endless succession of parasitism which once drove Jonathan Swift to write:

> . . . a flea
> Has smaller fleas that on him prey
> And these have smaller still to bite 'em
> And so on *ad infinitum*.

Swift must have also appreciated that the purpose of every living organism is to survive and produce progeny which it can only do by parasitising other organisms and turning their substance into that of its own kind. Man's infectious diseases result from the invasion of parasites which are not yet biologically adapted to their human hosts and accordingly cause characteristic symptoms.

A parasite may be defined as an animal or plant which associates with a host of different species from which it derives food and sometimes shelter. Human beings are parasitic on other animals and on plants, and are themselves parasitised by organisms which are usually smaller than themselves. It has been the misfortune of Middle Africa that its people host a greater number of disease-bearing parasites than any other race. These pests have played a very large part in crippling the development of Africa and in limiting its contact with the remainder of the world.

Parasitism generally benefits the client and may harm the host, but the character of the parasites is constantly altering through the process of natural selection and in such a manner as to approach a condition of mutual tolerance with the host. Only thus can they maintain their food source. For the infecting organisms' ultimate objective is to attain a relationship called 'commensalism' ('eating at the same table') where neither parties are harmed by their relationship, and indeed both host and client may benefit from it.

An example of commensalism in Africa occurs in the relationship between a buffalo and an ox-picker bird. The latter spends most of its time riding on the buffalo's back which supplies it with a home and food in the shape of ticks; in return the bird removes harmful scabs from its host's hide and warns it of approaching danger by creating a disturbance as it flies away. Symbiosis is a similar relationship, but one of the partners is unable to live alone.

The parasites of man may be described as either internal or external according to whether they live inside or outside the host's body. Thus worms are internal parasites and fleas are external ones. The internal parasites gain entry to their host either through the mouth, lungs, skin and (rarely) the anus. Parasites are spoken of as 'aberrant' when they stray from their normal venue in the host.

When considering parasitism it is important to stress again that the client always strives to obtain a stable relationship with its host so that it may continue to provide nourishment and shelter. The goal of all parasites then is commensalism through evolutionary change resulting in diminution of its virulence or increased human resistance to it following long exposure to its infection. In consequence the severity of human infection tends to diminish. Thus that of scarlet fever has greatly declined during the past few decades.

The human illnesses of tropical Africa may now be seen as a struggle for survival between mankind and whole regiments of predatory, pathogenic organisms which are so tiny that they went unrecognised until the invention of the microscope allowed scientists to explore the world of the infinitely small.

The most primitive animal parasites affecting man are single-celled protozoa which reproduce themselves by dividing into two clones. However more evolved organisms may undergo forms of sexual reproduction that increases the possibility of genetic variation through the mixing of different parental strains. In many cases two hosts are involved in a parasite's life cycle. The animal in which the parasite's fertilised eggs are produced is then referred to as the definitive host; that to which the parasite's larval phase is transmitted is termed the intermediate host. Thus in bilharzia, the snail acts as intermediate host while man is the definitive host.

Many human parasites boast a longer lineage than their hosts. Mosquitoes for instance have been found preserved in fossil rock more than thirty million years old. Man, it seems, inherited some of his present parasites – mosquitoes, malaria parasites, lice, tapeworms and roundworms – from his hominid ancestors.

Human beings have become adapted to animal parasitism
in several ways, although generally less effectively than to
invasion by bacteria and viruses. The most common response is inflammation which represents an attempt at
physical destruction of the parasitic invader through ingestion by white blood cells, a process termed phagocytosis.
A different reaction attempts to wall off the parasite by the
thickening of tissues, but this fibrosis may lead to surgical
complications and even to cancer. In addition, the body
defends itself against parasites by the production of antibodies which are directed either at the physical destruction
of the invaders or the neutralisation of their toxins.

The production of immunity is a vastly complex subject,
but because of its importance in limiting tropical diseases it
must be briefly considered here. Immunity may be natural
or acquired, and absolute or relative. Africans living in
endemic malarial areas acquire resistance towards the most
dangerous form of the disease. Thus over many centuries
those African groups which were highly susceptible to
malaria toxins died off; the surviving members of a population were selected from stock which happened to possess a
high natural immunity to the disease.

Some Africans possess an inherited trait which also protects them from malaria: in this condition, called sickle-
aemia, the red pigment of the blood cells is abnormal. The
red blood cells in consequence rupture when the malaria
parasites enter them and expose the parasites to destruction
by the white blood cells. But this condition is unusual, and
generally human immunity to the disease results from a
capacity, following ancestral exposure to malaria, to produce proteins which specifically neutralise the harmful
products of the infecting organism. In the same way sleeping sickness in an endemic area is a relatively mild disease
among its African population, but if the disease is carried to
a virgin community which lacks immunity, it will run an
acute and usually fatal course. Sometimes a tropical disease

of viral origin will, in an endemic area, be mild in children. An example is yellow fever: where endemic it will affect a high proportion of the local children who, because of inherited protective antibodies, will experience only a mild illness and thereafter enjoy lifelong acquired immunity to the disease. But strangers entering the region succumb to a severe illness. Thus Negroes living in America are highly susceptible to yellow fever, whereas their kin in West Africa enjoy a high immunity.

Systematic attempts at eliminating tropical disease from Africa began towards the end of the nineteenth century and provide us with a story of immense human effort and remarkable human courage. The task was particularly formidable because Africa's animal parasites are far from being elementary or degenerate organisms. They are refined and aggressive, and among the most specialised forms of life on earth. These primitive organisms have succeeded in overcoming the enormous problems entailed in reaching a required position in the body of a specific host. They accomplish this by the use of an inherited instinct which seems as wonderful as human intelligence. Parasite life appears to be governed by some mysterious power that is far beyond our understanding. It is operated by a separated group-soul which directs each organism into a definitive plan that the individual parasite then executes step by step. If a single stage is omitted, the cycle is broken. Although man has transmitted only a few acquired memories (like suckling) to his progeny, these lowly parasitic protozoa, flukes and worms are born with instincts which allow them to seek out their specific hosts and then find a way within their bodies to their allotted target.

Some idea of the marvel of parasitism is provided by the study of the pilgrimage undertaken by the hookworm larva into man's lower gut. The adult worms are greyish-white, measure about a centimetre in length, and their heads are armed with cutting teeth. They inhabit man's small intestine, attaching themselves to its mucous membrane by their teeth and suckers. There they live for several years sucking blood from their human hosts.

The host exhibits no symptoms until he harbours more than fifty worms. The parasite load may, however, run into thousands and causes anaemia, abdominal pain, diarrhoea and increasing lethargy; the anaemia may become so severe as to cause dropsy and heart failure.

An estimated 457 million people in the world are believed to suffer from hookworm infestation, and the number is increasing. It is widespread in its original home of tropical Africa and has been exported to many other parts of the world. Surveys in some parts of sub-Saharan Africa have shown a ninety-one per cent infestation rate. Treatment with vermifuges is fortunately both cheap and effective. Protection can be obtained simply by wearing shoes and the provision of adequate latrines. The early Israelites followed sanitary instructions laid down in Deuteronomy (XXIII, 2–3), thus escaping the infection, and owed much of their ascendency to this.

The worms live in the human body attached to the mucous membrane of the small intestine, and only shift their position to copulate. After fertilisation the female worm discharges about thirty thousand eggs a day. Providing these are excreted onto warm moist ground, the eggs hatch out into larvae which feed voraciously on any faecal matter nearby, at the same time undergoing two separate moults to accommodate their increasing size. The larvae rarely move more than ten centimetres from their point of deposit.

The survival of the mature larvae depends entirely on contact with a bare-footed person, whose skin they are able to penetrate. Having bored through the skin of the foot, itself a remarkable exercise, the larvae enter a blood vessel in the foot and are passively carried in the blood stream through the heart to the lungs. Here the homing urge, one of the strongest of all the physiological instincts, compels the infant worms to penetrate the capillary walls of the blood vessels in the lungs and enter their air vesicles. The host may react to the irritation of their passage by coughing, but the majority of the worms survive to crawl up the human bronchi and trachea, miraculously without producing any provocative stimulus to cause further expectoration; as the larvae then crawls over the extremely sensitive tissues of the human larynx, they presumably secrete some local anaesthetic to inhibit the cough reflex. Instinct next directs the parasites to crawl into the host's pharynx, where they are swallowed and so reach the human stomach, from whose acid secretions they are somehow protected. The infant worms have now only a short journey to their destined resting place in man's small intestine (which surface recognition systems enable them to identity). This takes two days. It is, however, several weeks later that the worms may mature and lay eggs.

This migration of the hookworm is relatively simple compared with those of man's other animal parasites. Yet the wonder of parasitic cycles is sustained by enormous wastage. Of the thirty thousand eggs passed each day by a single pregnant hookworm, only a very small proportion will produce larvae which find a person to parasitize. Even these will be at considerable risk during the journey which follows through the human body.

But nature is ever prodigal with the individual units of animals' reproductory mechanism, since it employs wastage to obtain a wide genetic mix. The expenditure is well demonstrated in the human male, for only a minute fraction of the immense number of spermatazoa produced will find a human egg to fertilize. Yet such is the harmony of nature that this extravagant mechanism keeps a race viable, provided only that the external environment does not change too rapidly.

3

Africa's Encounter with Europe

WE NEVER REALLY got over our shock at Kachindomoto, and for years afterwards pondered the possible events which might have precipitated the appalling infirmity of Africa which had first been demonstrated to us in that lakeside village. Only gradually did we appreciate that the earlier good health of the African people had depended on population stasis and their established immunity to local diseases.

The population density of Black Africa during historical times was much lower than those of Europe and Asia, and most of its people lived in small communities which were virtually isolated from each other through lack of communications; their villages were surrounded by a huge wilderness which few had either reason or inclination to explore.

For thousands of years the inhabitants of these communities had been exposed to the same disease-bearing organisms to which they have developed or inherited countervailing immunities. They may not have achieved perfect accommodation with their parasites but many centuries of selective processes had created a crude form of tolerance between them which came close to commensalism.

To a lesser degree the inhabitants of Old Africa were protected by cultural responses to suspected dangers. People learned where possible to avoid polluted water or bush which harboured tsetse flies. Even trading patterns evolved which required minimal contact with strangers of whom the Africans were ever suspicious: the people of one village would lay out their goods for sale at a recognised boundary and then withdraw; the others would then display wares of approximately the same value before retreating; bargaining would continue in this fashion until the price was right. The whole exercise was thus completed without the principals meeting. It is interesting to note that in England during the plague of 1665–6 people responded to hazards of disease in similar fashion: they took their market produce to the boundary of afflicted communities whose people came later to collect the food, leaving their money behind.

The diseases among the secluded African communities were thus generally endemic and not epidemic in nature, and since so few people lived in each settlement they could not sustain the bacterial and viral infections of more crowded communities which require rapid passage from person to person if the germs are to survive.

But inevitably the seclusion of the African communities was broken from time to time by the arrival of strangers escaping from drought, infections, or danger and bringing with them disease against which the settled people had no immunity; at the same time the newcomers encountered previously unknown germs to which they were vulnerable; both groups went down with infections that were often fatal.

Accordingly for many centuries the medical pattern of disease in tropical Africa was an irregular one. It showed small transient pockets of disease wherever people had become infected by new pathogenic micro-organisms which had been carried to them by the ebb and flow of internal migration. Most of these old disasters are long forgotten, but a few are still remembered in folklore or were recorded by Arab travellers in West Africa.

The anonymity which had lain over tropical Africa for so long was finally broken down during the middle of the fifteenth century when Portuguese mariners ventured down its Atlantic coastline and briefly went ashore to kidnap some of the inhabitants to carry back for sale in Lagos. With this first encounter with Europe, sub-Saharan Africa was launched into the modern world, and the seclusion which for so long had safeguarded the health of its people was increasingly disrupted as the Atlantic slave trade got under way.

The slave trade on the west coast reached its peak during the first half of the nineteenth century, and it greatly increased the population movement and incidence of disease throughout western Africa. An estimated fourteen million Africans were transported across the Atlantic by the slavers and a far larger number were uprooted from their homes. Yet there are grounds for believing that the population loss to the trade and the spread of disease were largely off-set by a natural increase in the population during this same period, due to a marked improvement of the Africans' diet. For the slavers took pains to carry back New World crops to Africa as well as Europe, and it became common practice for them to plant maize and other nutritious crops near the embarkation points on the slave coast to feed the captives during the Atlantic crossing. The cultivation of maize spread rapidly throughout Africa and it is known to have become well established in the Congo basin and Angola by 1543. As maize was a far more nourishing diet than millet and cassava, the population expanded during this chaotic period.

Many events combined with the Atlantic slave trade to destabilise Black Africa following its first encounter with white men, and we may briefly consider them here before turning to examine the diseases prevalent in the sub-continent before the impact of Europe became more wounding and finally disastrous.

Some scholars have suggested that the conquest of the powerful Songhai state by Moroccan soldiers in 1589 was the fatal stimulus which led to the decline of Middle Africa. Certainly the destruction of this empire was followed by dynastic quarrels and wars between successor states which unleashed hordes of refugees and brought them into unfamiliar disease environments.

The Arab slave trade also played an important part in disrupting the earlier isolation of the Africans. Since the beginning of the Christian era Arabs from Muscat and Oman had raided East Africa for slaves but the traffic gained momentum during the 1840s after the abolition of the Atlantic trade and the Arabs' occupation of the convenient base of Zanzibar within striking distance of the coast. The Arab man-hunt now, for the first time, began to penetrate far inland reaching the Great Lakes of the interior and the upper Congo, and even trespassing upon the old hunting ground of the Atlantic trade.

European travellers in East and Central Africa during the height of the Arab incursions were horrified by the slavers' wanton cruelty. Verney Lovett Cameron, who led the Livingstone Relief Expedition into Africa during 1873, estimated that in order to deliver five thousand slaves at the coast, six times that numbers of Africans were killed by the slavers and a hundred villages devastated. Inevitably the number of refugees increased until, thanks to the efforts of the British government, the eastern slave trade virtually ended in 1875, but only after it had broken up the ancient African way of life in an enormous area of the continent.

Different incursions added to the general demoralisation and dispersal of isolated rural clans. Thus Portuguese intervention in West Africa led to continuous fighting in the Congo basin between 1545 and 1576, and ushered in a hundred years of war in Angola. Similarly the increasing power of Ashanti tribesmen sent them raiding to the coast at least five times between 1806 and 1874. Unprecedented contacts between alien people also followed the militant expansion of the Zulus under Chaka after 1820 which set hordes of fugitives and marauding impis moving northwards as far as the Great Lakes. Only a few years later the thrust of Afrikaner trekkers towards the Limpopo likewise caused whole tribes to leave their homelands and seek safety in Central Africa. One tribe, the Makololo thus set in motion, provides a good example of the danger of entering a strange disease environment. Under Zulu pressure the Makololo fled from their homeland in the Orange Free State to the Zambezi Valley. There they fought and en- slaved the far more numerous Barotse. But within two generations the Makololo had become so weakened by malaria, to which their new subjects had long enjoyed immunity, that their power declined and the Barotse were able to reassert control over the valley. Conquerors often carry allies with them in the shape of new diseases; the Makololo experience shows that the reverse may also occur.

An utterly different destablising element of the old African way of life emerged when vast numbers of guns were brought into Africa by entrepreneurs and legitimate merchants following the abolition of the Atlantic slave trade. During the American Civil War breech-loading rifles had come into general use, making huge numbers of flint- lock muskets and percussion guns suddenly obsolete. They were eagerly accepted by African chiefs for trade goods such as timber, gum (for confectionery), palm oil, gold, hides, ivory and beeswax. Large quantities of ancient muskets thus poured into Africa: fifteen thousand were sold in Maputo alone during 1875 and a million are esti- mated to have reached German East Africa (now Tanzania) during the period 1885–1902.

These firearms inevitably led to tribal wars as chiefs used them to help extend their domains. In place of the old static communities dwelling peacefully in Black Africa the con- tinent became filled with still more people on the move, bent on armed forays or flight, all of them exchanging their germs with other communities and extending the boun- daries of disease in tropical Africa.

The slave traders on the Guinea Coast were among the first to describe the prevalent diseases among the Africans living there, for they conducted rough medical examin- ations of the captives brought in before buying them. They reported a high incidence of malaria, yaws, guinea worm infestation, dysentery and eye infections; filariasis, sleeping sickness and yellow fever were also frequently seen. All these infections were soon introduced into the New World. The slavers were also disturbed by a disease which they quaintly named 'the vice'. Its only symptom was earth eating which we now know was caused by hookworm infestation. They treated 'the vice' with doses of white lead, today a common ingredient of paints; this inevitably caused abdominal pain without diarrhoea which, in their queer jargon, was accordingly known to the slaves as 'dry belly ache.'

Mungo Park, who visited the Niger basin twice between 1796 and 1805, had undergone a medical training and he also left an account of the diseases he encountered in Africa. Malaria, he wrote, was very common though its symptoms were mild among African adults; he thought it followed exposure to night dew. Park also noted a high frequency of yaws, elephantiasis due to filarial infection, guinea worm infestation, yellow fever and advanced leprosy. Dysentery, comparatively uncommon among adult Africans, nevertheless greatly harassed white men on the coast. Park also saw many cases of gonorrhoea but not a single one of syphilis. He was impressed by the way the Africans opened abscesses with a cautery in the form of a red hot spear-head, and by their methods of dealing with inflammation by cupping: the large end of a bullock horn, he wrote, was placed over the affected area and its severed point partially sealed with beeswax; the air within the horn was then sharply inhaled by the attendant so as to create a near-vacuum, after which a tiny aperture in the wax was sealed with 'a skilful movement of the tongue'. In addition, he described the Africans' belief in the healing powers of fetishes which were named 'Mumbo Jumbo', an expression which he introduced into the English language.

Park recorded the occurrence of smallpox in West Africa too and believed that it had been carried there by infected Moors from across the Sahara. He did not come across measles, though it was reported from the same region during 1830.

David Livingstone made the largest contribution to our knowledge of diseases in sub-Saharan Africa during his travels through the continent from 1841–73. He found syphilis to be rare and seen only in men and women of mixed blood, but he noted a similar disease which was probably yaws. Dysentery, however, was common among the people during the rains, apparently of the amoebic type since it was frequently associated with liver abscess. Pneumonia was prevalent during the African winters and Livingstone noted that smallpox and measles had both appeared on the continent in epidemic form about 1835 but had since 'vanished'. He was the first man to note the occurrence of haematuria (blood in the urine) among Africans in what was an early reference to bilharzia, and of a worm that wandered about in African patients' eyes; no doubt he had seen cases of filariasis.

Livingstone also wrote at length about tropical ulcers and noted signs of two deficiency diseases; scurvy and the dimness of vision affecting people who lived on a predominantly cereal diet. He remarked on the fever associated with ticks, marvelled at the prevalence of tapeworms in men and women and the absence in Africans of stones in the bladder and insanity – although subsequently mental disturbances were frequently noted among them. Pulmonary tuberculosis was rare among the people in Livingstone's time. He himself suffered repeatedly from malaria during his travels and attained some immunity to it; he was frequently bitten by tsetse flies without ill effect, though he knew that their bites were fatal to cattle.

Lovett Cameron, who crossed Central Africa during 1872–5, confirmed most of Livingstone's findings (including the fact that smallpox had 'swept through' the continent some decades earlier) though he seems to have seen more cases of leprosy. Both men praised the endurance of their porters; Livingstone went so far as to compare the stamina of the Makololo to that of the argonauts, and he does not give the impression of the Africans being a particularly sickly race. Yet only a few years after his death in 1873, the picture had changed. Thus, Sir Harry Johnston who began his long service in Africa during 1883 came to the conclusion that its people were no more than a 'hive of gangrenous germs'. Stanley too recognised a high morbidity among the Africans during his long march to relieve Emin Pasha which began in 1887. In modern Zaire he left a rearguard of five Englishmen behind in a staging camp together with two hundred and sixty of his porters. There, according to one of the officers, the Africans died off 'like rotten sheep', and on Stanley's return fourteen months later only one European and sixty surviving porters were there to meet him.

At Kachindomoto, some fifty years afterwards, we realised that 'something dreadful had happened to rural Africa' during the past century and we had some evidence that the main calamity had begun just before or during the early 1880s.

4

A Victory for Empiricism

DURING THE EARLIER YEARS of the encounter between
Europe and Africa which led up to the main contact in the
1880s, a slowly increasing number of white men came out to
live in tropical Africa. To begin with the majority were
either slave traders who established themselves along the
Guinea Coast, or Portuguese colonists sent out to Angola
and Mozambique. The number of Europeans on the coast
subsequently grew when soldiers were posted to the string
of forts established at strategic points by the maritime
powers to protect their trading interests. Later on sailors of
the Royal Navy serving in the anti-slavery patrols were also
based on harbours along the slave coasts following the abolition of the British slave trade in 1807. These expatriates
were presently followed to Africa by explorers and a growing number of missionaries. All of them suffered far more
than their black neighbours from tropical diseases, since
they lacked the latters' higher degree of immunity to local
infections.

Indeed the European mortality was appallingly high and
most of it was caused by malaria. During the eighteenth
century it was estimated that between twenty-five and
seventy-five per cent of white newcomers would die during
their first year on the Guinea Coast. A hundred years later
the mortality rate had not improved. Between 1804 and
1825 over sixty per cent of the men sent out by the Church
Missionary Society to West Africa succumbed to disease.
The figures for local military garrisons were even more
fearful: out of one unit numbering one thousand five
hundred and sixty-eight soldiers which was stationed on the
coast between 1822 and 1830, one thousand two hundred

and ninety-eight died there from 'climatic fevers' while
another one hundred and twenty-five perished during the
voyage home; half the survivors subsequently succumbed to
tropical disease in England, and only fifty-seven were finally
discharged as fit. The mortality among the crews of the
Royal Navy's anti-slavery patrol off the Guinea Coast was so
high that the sailors spoke of it as 'the coffin squadron',
while those based on Bathurst knew the port as 'Half Die'.
The European slavers on captured ships were sometimes
landed on the coast; of fifty men so marooned during 1841,
forty died from fever within three months.

The Europeans were well aware that the Africans on the
coast were comparatively free from the diseases which
struck themselves down in such numbers. No-one was able
to account for their relative immunity from fever, though it
was feared that it might be a case of the survival of the fittest
which raised worrying thoughts that the whites in the world
might one day be replaced by better endowed blacks. It was
more comforting to conclude that the Africans' greater
facility for sweating threw off noxious humors from the
blood, but this theory had to be abandoned after a group of
philanthropists settled escaped slaves from America at
Freetown in Sierra Leone, for these newcomers promptly
went down with fevers as severe as those suffered by the
Europeans.

It was not surprising then that the Guinea Coast became
known as the white man's grave. The death rate there was
far higher than in the tropical outposts of India, Batavia and
the West Indies, for not only did the coast harbour such
killing diseases as malaria, sleeping sickness and yellow
fever, but it lacked nearby salubrious stations where con-
valescents might recuperate. The best that could be done
for the sick was to ship them off to places like Ascension
Island where today it is a moving experience to walk about
the beaches among the rounded stones that mark the last
resting places of those who perished from the infections of
nearby Africa.

The British explorers of West Africa fared no better than the slave merchants, soldiers and missionaries. Of the forty men who made up Mungo Park's second expedition to the Niger in 1805, not one returned to England: six were killed; the remainder died from malaria or dysentery.

The toll among European explorers continued. When a second British sortie to the Niger under a Captain Peddie followed in Park's tracks, a third of his men died before he turned back to the coast. Soon afterwards Commander Tuckey RN pioneered a river route up the Congo but only after losing nearly half his crew from fever, although their deaths were officially attributed to 'drinking Congo water'.

Then in 1841 the first official British Niger expedition set out for West Africa. It was intended that the expedition proceed up the river in three boats and form a permanent settlement at Lokosa from which the blessings of civilisation and Christianity might be dispensed to the surrounding country. The expedition collapsed when fever struck the ships. Forty-two white men died from malaria out of a complement of one hundred and forty-five. Yet of the one hundred and fifty-eight locally recruited Africans on board, only eleven developed fever, and all survived. It was a remarkable demonstration of the adult African's immunity to his particular brand of malaria.

The losses from the Niger expedition both horrified the British public and stimulated interest in malaria. The disease was known to be an ancient one, but its cause was quite unknown and many more years would pass before it was recognised to be due to a blood parasite of man which it is believed also affected the early hominids. Probably the human parasite evolved from simple coccidial protozoa present in the lower bowel of man's distant ancestors. These then accidentally entered the host's blood stream and succeeded in adapting to life in their new environment. Next their hominid and human hosts were parasitised by mosquitoes, and another adaptation allowed the blood parasites to spend part of their lives in these insect hosts. In them they underwent a form of sexual reproduction which carried valuable genetic advantages.

In this way man became the host to both malaria parasites and female mosquitoes which require a human blood feed before they can lay fertilised eggs. Over three thousand species of mosquito are known and the anopheline species, of which there are more than a hundred strains, includes the several transmitters of human malaria. Infestation of mosquitoes by malarial parasites does them no harm; together they have entered into a state of mutual tolerance. The female anopheline mosquito behaves like a vampire in sucking human blood, but the male insect is a mild-mannered vegetarian which obtains most of its food from the nectar of flowers.

In a single meal the female mosquito ingests one to two millilitres of blood, which is about two-and-a-half times her own weight. If this feed contains malaria parasites, some will undergo fertilisation, reproduction and growth within the insect's body until they are ready to be injected into a new human host. They are then transmitted in saliva during the mosquito's biting process.

The symptoms of malaria have remained unchanged since they were first described over two thousand years ago. This contrasts with other diseases whose features have varied greatly over the centuries. Thus the manifestations of scarlet fever have altered within living memory while the once dreaded sweating sickness has completely disappeared.

Malaria was well known in ancient Greece. Sir Ronald Ross believed that the disease appeared there about 500 BC, perhaps introduced by infected slaves, and was largely responsible for the country's subsequent decadence. Hippocrates (460–370 BC) wrote an admirable description of its manifestations. He also recognised its variety of forms; these include quotidian or daily fever, and tertian fever which occurs on alternate days. Hippocrates believed malaria to be caused by drinking stagnant water. Columella (c.

AD 116), however, thought it came from germs present in marshy ground, and he suspected that the infection was transmitted by gnats and mosquitoes. Alexander the Great was one of malaria's victims.

Rome was so subject to epidemics of malaria that a goddess of fever, *Dei Febris*, was worshipped for her power to cure the disease, and the fall of the empire was said to have been due to the illness's debilitating effect on its citizens. At least three emperors, Hadrian, Vespasian and Titus, are believed to have died from it. St Augustine is said to have suffered from malaria contracted on the road from Rome to Ostia when carrying Christianity to Britain.

Malaria was widespread throughout medieval Europe, and only died out after land reclamation and improved drainage did away with mosquitoes. It has also been suggested that an increase in animal husbandry led to mosquitoes gaining a preference for cows's blood and turned to biting them rather than men. In addition the building of well-lit and ventilated houses proved inhospitable to them. Malaria was especially common in the fenlands of England and the marshy ground of the Thames Valley. Both James I and Oliver Cromwell died from the disease. Malaria finally disappeared from London in 1859 after the building of the Thames Embankment. Before this date five per cent of admissions to St Thomas' Hospital were due to it.

In parts of Africa the association of fever with mosquitoes was recognised by the inhabitants, and in one area the name 'mbu' was applied to both the insect and the disease it caused. In medieval Europe weird beliefs existed regarding its origin. Planets and comets were said to rain down a fever-poison on the earth; elsewhere electrical storms were held responsible; even the angle of the sun's rays in the tropics was incriminated. Only gradually was the association of the disease with marshy ground accepted, and efforts to understand the fever became concentrated on what was called the 'miasmatic theory'. This submitted that swamp air contained chemical poisons which had been freed from rotting wood. The hypothesis died hard. As late as 1881 mission houses on the shores of Lake Malawi were built to face inland to avoid 'miasmata' being blown in over the water, while double story buildings were favoured since it was believed that the miasma did not rise far above ground level. Although as early as 1848, a Dr Josia Nott of Mobile, Alabama, wrote an article suggesting that malaria was transmitted by mosquitoes, his suggestion was ignored. Instead most other nineteenth-century appreciations of the cause of malaria in Africa were as bizarre as the medieval theories. Thus we find the talented traveller Winwood Reade gravely asserting during the 1850s that when dew fell on ships' decks before sunrise, it produced small insects resembling lizards, toads and serpents which carried the fever, and he added that they particularly sought out human victims of fair complexion who were prone to drunkenness, 'strumous habits' and lethargic dispositions.

Treatment for malaria did not alter in Europe for centuries. Despite their futility, the old methods of therapy continued to be employed; the lying in steam baths, cold dips in the sea, application of blisters, the swallowing of strychnine, arsenic and calomel in heroic doses, and the application of leeches, the last so frequently used that they gave their name to medical practitioners. Blood-letting, however, was the most favoured remedy for fever; this was effected by opening a vein in the arm and bandaging it tightly when sufficient blood had been allowed to drip into a bowl. Usually about sixteen ounces (450 ml) of blood were withdrawn, but twice this amount was sometimes taken and in extreme cases as much as a hundred ounces has been recorded which is about half the blood content of an adult. It was not surprising that when effective quinine therapy came into use, the benefits which resulted were partly ascribed to the abandonment of the older barbarous methods of treatment. Preventive measures against malaria, however, were generally limited to wearing linen bags around the neck containing garlic and camphor, and using crude mosquito nets.

A growing appreciation of the association of 'the ague' with marshy ground led to it being given new names like marsh fever, river fever, paludal fever, bilious remittent fever and finally malaria, meaning 'bad air'. And a great break through in treatment, a triumph of empiricism, took place in 1640 with the acceptance of cinchona as a specific remedy for the disease.

The story of quinine begins in Peru, where Indians for centuries had known the beneficial use in fever of the bark of a tree named *Myroxylon*. Legend insists that they were introduced to its effects by watching pumas chewing the tree when they were ill. The Indians, who called the bark 'kina' or even 'kina-kina', meaning 'bark of barks', were in the habit of stripping it from trees and soaking it in water to make an infusion which was taken by mouth. Some time after the Spanish Conquest, a converted Indian chief prescribed kina-kina for a Catholic missionary suffering from fever, and with such good effect that the curative qualities of the 'Jesuit bark' presently became known throughout Spanish America.

According to a time-honoured tradition the bark was used to cure fever in the wife of the Viceroy of Peru, the Count de Chinchon, and the name of the illustrious patient was given to it. By mischance the 'H' was omitted and it became known as cinchona. The legend is attractive but more probably the name was in fact derived from the Peruvian 'kina-kina'.

The miraculous drug was soon introduced into Europe by the Jesuits who gave it freely to the poor but charged its weight in gold to the wealthy. The reputation of cinchona increased after its administration cured the Archduke Leopold of ague in 1653. A physician, Richard Talbor, then successfully prescribed it for Charles II when he went down with malaria. Talbor was later knighted by his royal patient and made a fortune prescribing his mixture of the bark in wine. He died in 1681 and lies buried in Trinity Church, Cambridge.

Zealous Protestants looked askance at the virtues of the Jesuit bark and it was denied Oliver Cromwell when he lay dying of malaria. Other rulers were more fortunate and it is even recorded that an emperor of China was successfully treated with cinchona. The famous physician, Sir Thomas Sydenham (1624–89) was active in popularising the drug in Britain. To obtain a cure he measured thirty-two grams of the bark into two pints of wine; this was then divided into twelve doses and taken every four hours.

Cinchona was also given prophylactically but reports of its efficacy differed. For every sample of the bark varied markedly in potency, and it was always difficult to ensure that the vile tasting infusions of the bark were in fact swallowed by chary patients – especially the suspicious soldiers of the African garrisons. Certainly cinchona served the Niger expedition of 1841 badly, and became discredited for some time as a result. Perhaps its failure was due to the poor quality of the bark or because its distribution was inadequately supervised, factors which had led to previous ups and downs in the drug's popularity.

Fortunately the use of cinchona alkaloids was placed on a more rational basis when two French pharmacists succeeded in isolating the alkaloids of quinine from the bark, by distillation and crystallisation. After 1820 it thus became possible to prescribe quinine powder in known strength, and it was generally available after 1854 when Dutch settlers established cinchona plantations in Java and developed an extensive export trade.

David Livingstone was convinced of the efficacy of quinine treatment for malaria during 1850 when he cured two of his children who had gone down with the fever. Thereafter he became a firm advocate of quinine therapy, devising a compound tablet which combined it with rhubarb, calomel and jalap. These became known as 'Livingstone Rousers' and were widely used.

Quinine admittedly suffered from several disadvantages. No one had the faintest idea of how the drug worked, it possessed a bitter taste, deafness followed prolonged use, and it sometimes induced nausea and vomiting which might seriously detract from its therapeutic effect (Mrs Livingstone was one of many who died because she could not hold down her tablets). In addition the drug had some mysterious association with the onset of the dreaded blackwater fever which occasionally complicated malaria. This complication was once one of the most common causes of death among expatriates in Africa. Its cause is still unknown but is somehow related to taking irregular doses of prophylactic quinine. 'Blackwater' is now rarely seen following the introduction of synthetic anti-malaria drugs.

Only four years after Livingtstone's conversion to quinine, a second Niger expedition proceeded to demonstrate the drug's effectiveness. Command of this 1854 expedition devolved on a Dr W.B. Baikie. He had fortunately already learned of the success attending the disciplined administration of quinine to British troops who had landed in the malarial Danube delta on their way to fight the Russians in the Crimea. Baikie consequently instituted a similar regime on the Niger, and presently returned triumphantly to England without having lost a single man. Unfortunately Baikie had not appreciated that certain types of malaria may relapse long after leaving an endemic area, and he died on his way home from a second expedition because he stopped taking quinine immediately after leaving the coast.

The good results from quinine prophylaxis was confirmed by Livingstone during the Zambezi Expedition of 1858–64. When in malarial areas he distributed quinine regularly to his companions and reported in glowing terms on its efficacy. This success was widely publicised and another milestone in African history had been passed, for at last it was possible for Europeans to enter the dark continent and live there in comparative freedom from its greatest danger. They could now compete with Arab travellers

whose apparant resistance to malaria had long been puzz-
ling. In fact most of the so-called Arabs who roamed
through eastern Africa were of mixed blood and had inherited their African forebears' immunity. In addition their
flowing robes and headwear tended to limit access of mosquitoes to their bodies.

Realisation of the efficacy of quinine coincided with the
introduction of the breech-loading rifle which gave white
men increased confidence in their ability to survive the
other threats they might meet in Africa. From now on the
exploration of the continent proceeded apace, with interest
moving away from the Guinea coast to the country lying to
the east of the great Rift Valley.

Several complementary factors are responsible for this
shift of interest. The Royal Navy had recently gained control of the Indian Ocean as well as the Atlantic, and the use
of the overland Suez route to India led to the establishment
of military stations at Aden, Socotra and Karachi. After
Captain W.F. Owen RN successfully completed a survey of
the eastern coast in 1823, and Zanzibar became recognised
as an unexpectedly convenient jumping off place for expeditions of exploration, it was found that the east African
plateau offered attractions notably absent on the Guinea
coast. For tropical Africa may be divided into two portions
by an imaginary line on the map joining Angola to Ethiopia.
The ground to the north of this line mainly comprises
sedimentary basins with land rising no more than 600 metres
above sea level. Almost all of the country south of this line,
however, rises above 1,000 metres; even the surface of Lake
Victoria is 1,130 metres above sea level. Accordingly the
climate of East Africa was far better than on the west coast,
even stimulating. The great plains of the eastern savannah
were healthy, and immense herds of game roamed them,
providing magnificent sport for adventurers. News too had
reached England of the discovery by German missionaries
of two snow-capped mountains in Kenya and Tanzania, and
rumours from up country suggested that the Ancients'

accounts of a great lake in the interior might well prove true; if so this would provide easy navigation through much of the hinterland. Then, in 1857, David Livingstone caught the imagination of the British public with an account of his exploration of East Central Africa which he had approached from the south, and where he found salubrious areas suitable for European settlement. His book, *Missionary Travels*, ended with an irresistible call to his countryman to send out civilising missions into the African interior. His piteous death among the swamps of Lake Bengweulu sixteen years later only added to this appeal.

Other factors quickened interest in the eastern part of the continent. The government of India, conscious of the area's strategic importance encouraged army officers to spend their leaves there. This stimulus resulted in the appearance of a new breed of explorers. They were often professional soldiers, men of substance, blatantly British, full of confidence and far better able than their predecessors to guard themselves against the perils of Africa. They not only carried life-saving quinine and guns, but were fitted out too with other modern manufactures, ranging from tinned food to inflatable rubber boats. Even protection against rain was provided by new-fangled macintoshes.

Though some of the new explorers still made rough sketches of African scenes (which would presently be copied by wood engravers for the inevitable travelogues), the newly invented camera became increasingly useful in the search for authenticity. Fold-up beds and chairs provided for the travellers' comfort in the bush, and their clothing was carried in insect-proof tin boxes (which their porters believed in fact contained spare, fold-up Europeans ready to be assembled in an emergency). In any case, expeditions to East Africa were far less perilous and much more profitable than ventures to the west coast. There was a very good chance that the explorers who set off from Zanzibar would eventually return home safely with loads of ivory and with every intention of setting down their adventures in leather-bound volumes which were assured of good sales to a public consumed with curiosity for Africa.

With them, in increasing numbers, missionaries were beginning to enter what they termed 'darkest Africa'. Livingstone had inspired a new era of philanthropic endeavour in the continent. East Africa, even more than the west coast became a place of atonement for the slave trade, a place where missionaries could test God's powers of protection. Here in the 'dark continent' they hoped to make journeys which might be attended by miracles and even martyrdom. The work of these dedicated men of God was every bit as important in opening up the continent as that of the explorers. They were fit successors to the Portuguese missionaries who had first carried Christianity to the Congo two centuries earlier. These priests were men of marvellous fortitude, enthusiasm and endurance. They nourished a remarkable theory that, to survive, they must exhaust their veins of European blood, and allow it to be replaced by the blood of Africa. Accordingly they repeatedly bled and purged themselves; one monk named Carli was bled ninety times. Their mortality rate was appalling but the memory of their sacrifice lingered among the Africans for centuries.

But the later generation of missionaries rarely figured in the headlines; glamour instead mantled the lay explorers of eastern Africa. The exploits of the sardonic Burton and unfortunate Speke were eagerly followed by the public after their arrival at Lake Tanganyika in 1858, and Speke presently showed that the fabled sea of Ujiji was in fact only one lake among several. For shortly afterwards Speke and Grant revealed Lake Victoria to be the true source of the Nile, Livingstone reached Nyasa, and Samuel Baker, accompanied by his future wife, found another inland sea, Lake Albert. After that Stanley was most often in the news. Having found Livingstone at Ujiji, Stanley followed the Lualaba to the west and demonstrated that it was in fact the Congo. There remained a few more geographical gaps to fill, but within a remarkably short time, a dozen men made sure that by 1880 nearly all the hinterland of East Africa had been explored.

By now these new explorers had become adept at discovering means to ensure their well-being in tropical Africa, and it is worthwhile here to pause briefly to study their methods since they played a part in allowing Europeans to open up the continent. Most of them carried a copy of Francis Galton's *Art of Travel*.* The book had been published by John Murray in 1855, and ran through eight editions, the last dated 1893. It contained all sorts of advice ranging from the proper handling of porters to the treatment of scorpion stings. Thus it usefully pointed out that when applying a tourniquet it was worth remembering that 'the main arteries follow much the same direction as the seams of the sleeves and trousers'. But Galton also sometimes misled his readers as when he advised explorers with a penchant for mountaineering to carry a cat with them, since these unfortunate animals acted as barometers and were invariably seized by convulsions precisely when they reached 13,000 feet.

Therapeutic approaches had altered too. Gone now was the habit of bleeding sick colleagues to 'restore a proper fluid balance in the body', and whereas Bristol ships at the beginning of the century had made do with medical chests containing only jalap, croton oil, calomel, and cinchona bark, by now quinine in tablets of known composition and strength was only one of the many drugs available to African pathfinders. Richard Lander's pharmacopoeia in 1832 already contained calomel, Epsom salts, Seidlitz powder, tartar emetic, citric acid (in lieu of lemon juice), sodium bicarbonate, blue pills, packets of Dr James' powder to encourage sweating, and two pints of opium. The explorers subsequently added Easton syrup to their list of

---

* Galton, after coming under the influence of his cousin Charles Darwin, founded the science of eugenics. He qualified as a doctor, explored Southern Africa and subsequently researched brilliantly into colour blindness and the use of finger prints for identification purposes.

patent medicines, together with Collis Browne's chloro-
dyne, Carter's Little Liver Pills, Cockle's antibilious tablets,
and a tin of Beecham's famous products. Thomas Baines
during the seventies appreciated the value of zinc sulphate
drops for conjunctivitis, and he used millboard for emergency splinting. Vast quantities of purges were carried too,
for it was considered to be a sovereign remedy for all
manner of illnesses affecting African porters. Diachylon
plasters were particularly favoured by their masters for
lumbago and happily the black camp followers discovered
they were also efficacious abortifacients.

Toothache remained a perennial problem among the
explorers, and sufferers were earnestly advised to push and
pull at the offending tooth until it was loose enough to
pull out with the fingers. Haemorrhage from a wound was
sternly staunched with a red-hot ramrod, gunpowder was
exploded on a snake bite to prevent the spread of venom,
and travellers learned to avoid chills by sleeping between
two large fires. In an emergency a charge of gunpowder in a
cup of warm water was known to be an effective emetic, wild
geranium root was advocated for dysentery, and an emul-
sion of male fern (to be found growing in ant-bear holes) was
known to be remedial in stomach upsets. Silver wire was
available for suturing wounds, and Galton shrewdly advised
that drugs be carried in zinc pill boxes with their names
embossed on both top and bottom in case the lids were
accidentally changed.

Although in quinine they now possessed a remedy for
malaria, there still remained considerable disagreement
among the explorers about the cause of the disease, and
more grotesque theories were advanced before the real
answer became known at the end of the nineteenth century.
Burton for instance ascribed fever to sleeping out in the
bright moonlight, while Stanley thought it was due to a
mysterious substance in the air called ozone. Livingstone
glimpsed the truth when he associated the disease with
'myriads of mosquitoes'. Others thought it might be due to

alcoholism, and missionaries sometimes even referred to fever as 'whiskyitis'. Certainly many newcomers to Africa were advised, with little noticeable effect, to avoid alcohol in any form, at least before sundown. Coffee and tea were recommended instead. Much later General Gordon had the best of both worlds by enjoying both of these beverages, while prudently lacing them with brandy. However, many of the old hands regarded whisky as the sovereign remedy for fever.

There were other changes too as the century drew towards its close. Norfolk jackets became almost *de rigeur* for white travellers in East Africa, and flannel was generally worn next to the skin. Umbrellas were long a popular item of equipment (the sunshade had yet to appear). Heavy boots, a size too large (to allow for swollen feet) were generally advised, and some men exchanged long trousers and socks for shorts (which came down well below the knees) and puttees. The benefits of citronella oil as a mosquito repellant were recognised and the use of mosquito nets became commonplace; drinking water was generally boiled after the 1870s, and presently the invention of porcelain filters and thermos flasks added to the travellers' safety and comfort.

After fever, the demon sun remained the white man's chief enemy in Africa. Sunstroke was greatly feared. It was to be avoided by wearing a preposterous coal-scuttle helmet made of white rubber or cork with a puggaree round the crown to give it style. Livingstone, however, had preferred a peaked cap but this never caught on, nor did Stanley's high-crowned hat with a ring of brass-lined holes to allow circulation of air round the head. More comely felt hats with a double brim (the terai) enjoyed a later vogue in Africa, but still the fear of sunstroke persisted. As late as the 1930s Schweitzer was busy warning his disciples that a ray of sunlight passing through a chink in the roof no larger than a florin might cause fatal brain haemorrhage if it touched on their heads. Cholera belts were worn by some men, others felt lost without their spine-pads. Later on dark glasses (Livingstone ordered a pair in London as early as 1848) were added to the tropical kit, and the products of Crosse and Blackwell came to occupy a place in travellers' lives almost as important as quinine.

The introduction of quinine in defined dosage and the experience gained in the eastern grasslands of Africa went far in making West Africa also safe for the white man, but still it was haunted by the spectre of witchcraft and mumbo jumbo which kept people away. Towards the end of last century even these fears were finally banished. A 'frail spinster', Mary Kingsley, played a notable part in disposing of them. This character from a Jane Austen novel travelled alone and safely through areas where previous explorers had fared so badly. She was well respected by the Africans who commonly addressed her as 'sir'. In 1897 Miss Kingsley described their country with a charming archness and presented the Africans as a friendly, helpful people who suffered cruelly from disease and poverty, and were greatly in need of European understanding and assistance. She successfully played down the danger of fever to prospective white visitors, advising them merely to 'take four grains of quinine every day and get some introduction to the Wesleyans: they are the only people on the coast who have got a hearse with feathers'. Her account removed the stigma from an apparently hostile land; the Guinea coast now finally lost its terrors, and the whole of Africa lay open to European penetration.

5

The Conquest of Africa

DURING THE 1870s, as the new-style explorers were un-
covering the secrets of East Africa, very few Africans had
actually encountered Europeans. Admittedly, white men
had lived for several hundred years on the Guinea Coast,
but their numbers never exceeded three thousand at a time.
In any case few of them survived the diseases of the coast for
long, and those who did become 'seasoned' made little
attempt to explore the continent's hinterland. Further
south the Portuguese colonists of Angola and Mozambique
were more enterprising. They established themselves in the
healthy highlands east of Luanda and in scattered stations
on the Zambezi. But the military expeditions they launched
into the interior withered away under the onslaught of
malaria and dysentery, while those few missionaries and
traders who gained a foothold in what is now Zimbabwe
were expelled before 1700.

Yet if only a small minority of the inhabitants of Black
Africa had in 1880 set eyes on a white face, within twenty
years they were to know Europeans far too well. For by then
the white men had imposed their rule over most of tropical
Africa during that remarkable burst of expansionist energy
which had been called the 'scramble for Africa'.

The scramble began quite suddenly. On looking back
afterwards, Lord Salisbury remembered that 'When I left
the Foreign Office in 1880, nobody thought much about
Africa. When I returned in 1885, the nations of Europe
were almost quarrelling with each other as to the various
portions of Africa south of the Sahara they could obtain.'
But already the dangers of competitive annexation had
been recognised, and towards the end of 1884 represent-

atives of fourteen European nations met in Berlin to find ways of settling their conflicting African claims before they led to war. Compromises were quickly reached and frock-coated statesmen joined each other in tracing frontier lines on their maps which carved up the continent in a manner that was without reference to history, geography or ethnic considerations.

Following this paper-partition of Africa, officials were sent out to take over the administration of the new African colonies, dependencies and protectorates. They were confident now of the efficacy of quinine in preventing and curing malaria, and already the death rate of Europeans on the Guinea coast had fallen by eighty per cent. Quinine was in plentiful supply and it had become the prime factor in allowing the white man's conquest of Black Africa. A secondary factor was his monopoly of modern guns.

The European powers were able to pick up huge parcels of undeveloped estate cheaply and at little risk from armed resistance; for now, thanks to the possession of new repeating rifles and machine guns, the power differential between Europe and Black Africa was greater than ever before, and it would not alter for the next seventy years.

Leopold I, king of the Belgians, was one of the first to appreciate the vulnerability and commercial opportunities of Africa. After failing to establish colonies in the Philippines and Borneo, he decided that he 'must lose no chance of winning a share of this magnificent cake of Africa'. For this purpose he enlisted the help of Henry Morton Stanley who had just completed his remarkable journey from the east coast of Africa to the heart of the continent, finally emerging in 1879 on its Atlantic coast. Stanley returned to Africa as the King's agent and on 13 June 1880 signed the first of a succession of treaties with bewildered chiefs which eventually handed over the sovereignty of two million square kilometres of land to be held as Leopold's personal fief. Competitive annexations increased after 1882. Germany laid claims to Togo, Cameroun, Tanganyika and gained a foothold in Namibia; Great Britain formalised her occupation of land on the Guinea Coast while the French established themselves in Dahomey and on the right bank of the Congo.

These were the great days of empire building, and it is remarkable how much of this was done by individuals acting on their own initiative. The example set by King Leopold was followed by Karl Peters, Cecil Rhodes, Frederick Lugard, Savergan de Brazza, George Goldie and several others, and their treaties were usually ratified by their governments.

Rapacity then was the main reason for the land grab in Africa, but other motives may be recognised. One was the question of national prestige. During the 1880s a delicate balance of power preserved the peace of Europe, but international rivalry could still find positive expression in the less sensitive colonial field. If one state acquired a useful block of land somewhere in the wet tropics, this gain would be quickly balanced by counter-annexations by other countries. It was like overtrumping during a game of cards. As always, Great Britain was concerned about the sea routes to India and to secure them she seized land round Mombasa and Berbera. Germany would then respond by proclaiming sovereignty over a place like Dar-es-Salaam while France took over another part of Central Africa. The chain reaction resulted in nearly all Black Africa coming under white rule by the end of the century.

Commercial interest in Europe welcomed these cheap conquests since they protected established trading patterns and initiated new ones. Thus a demand for ivory (to make billiard balls, piano keys, combs, knife handles and ornaments) at once drew the powers' attention to those parts of Africa which supported large herds of elephant. But less unlovely motives sometimes also led to annexations. Genuine concern existed about the breakdown of indigenous order and economic systems in Africa as its peoples became increasingly trapped in a cycle of tribal strife, disease and malnutrition during the years preceding the 'scramble'. The establishment of European rule, it was hoped, would bring back peace to the regions together with the blessings of civilisation and an opportunity of improving the people's health.

Yet a certain amount of hypocrisy also accompanied the conquest as the new administrators settled down sounding the note of 'governing to serve'. Leopold of Belgium struck an odious pose of acting as God's prefect when he set about exploiting the wealth and people of the Congo Free State, and the French did not sound entirely convincing when they spoke of their duty to spread Gallic culture among their new subjects.

But what perhaps was most remarkable about the European seizure of sub-Saharan Africa was that although the rudimentary health services that were set up recognised the mounting danger from sleeping sickness, there was little appreciation that the incidence of other diseases among the Africans also rose steeply following the conquest.

For the increased population movements which then occurred set epidemics raging across the continent. Some resulted from punitive expeditions to suppress risings which broke out across Africa as the people recovered from the first shock of conquest and resisted the imposition of unfamiliar laws and the hated hut tax. White officers would then lead columns of askaris followed by a swarm of porters across the continent on punitive expeditions living off the land, burning standing crops to crush resistance, and leaving a swathe of famine behind them. With them the soldiers also carried the germs of disease to virgin territories. Between 1890 and 1910 innumerable risings were put down in countries like Zimbabwe, Uganda, Sierra Leone, Somaliland (where the 'mad Mullah' kept the flame of rebellion alight until 1920), Nigeria, Tanzania (the 'Maji Maji' rebellion), and Namibia ('the Herero Rising'). These and the 1887 expedition mounted by Stanley to rescue Emin Pasha from the Equatoria province of the Sudan became particularly notorious for disseminating disease.

Forced labour, a feature of early colonial rule in Africa, was another factor in spreading infections. Thus the recruitment of labourers in the Congo Free State caused thousands of workers to abandon their villages to tap the natural rubber of the forests, and ships plying the elaborate tributary system of the Congo river carried their germs far across the continent.

The demand for migratory labour by mines as well as plantations also led to a high toll of disease among the workers and the people with whom they mixed. Men from Mozambique, Zimbabwe and Malawi took their diseases to the distant gold mines of Johannesburg and presently brought new strains of organisms back to their homelands. Others living in the Kenya highlands, who had no previous contact with malaria, were engaged to labour on harbour works in Mombasa and there died off at the appalling rate of one hundred and forty-five per thousand, while the death rate among labourers on the Congo-Océan railway was almost as high. Elsewhere the toll taken by the European demand for labour was scarcely less horrifying. Senegalese sent off to distant ground-nut plantations, and Tanzanian labour drafted to faraway sisal farms, all carried their special varieties of parasites to new communities, which in turn infected the foreign workers with the local diseases. The imposition of German authority in the Cameroons was likewise attended by disastrous medical consequences. In a single plantation between 1905 and 1906, six hundred and twenty-five labourers died out of a work force of under six thousand.

Resettlement programmes, labour migration, the extension of mining, the construction of dams and roads all dispersed diseases throughout tropical Africa. Later on labour would be concentrated in factories and for the first time set up ideal conditions for the spread of viral diseases like the common cold in many countries.

Even the imposition of efficient administrations on the

new colonies served to increase the number of people moving into unfamiliar disease environments. The Africans' new security led Dr George Maclean to note that 'with the suppression of tribal wars, the necessity for living in large villages for protection no longer existed. . . . It was now possible for a man and his family to go into the forest and start a remote settlement of their own.' Elsewhere a growing emphasis on export crops like coffee and groundnuts proved so remunerative to Africans that it led to a reduction in food production, while an increased oscillation of people back and forth from their villages to harvest rubber in changing areas of the Congo forests helped to spread disease on a previously unknown scale. Indeed, the very stability created by white men provided increasing opportunities for travelling along the roads and railways laid down by the governing powers. Other changes caused trouble: for instance, district commissioners, who commonly ruled areas the size of Wales, found it administratively convenient to concentrate scattered peasants under their charge into large villages where their activities were more easily supervised. Different communities were thus mixed together with disastrous consequences.

In 1890 an entirely unanticipated disaster added to the dissemination of disease: in that year rinderpest, a virus infection of cattle and game with a high mortality, raged through the East African savannah whose whole ecology depended on a delicate balance between man, cattle, game and the egregious tsetse fly. The infection is believed to have been introduced into Africa by cattle brought in for food and it soon spread throughout the continent.

When the rinderpest reached the savannah country, game and cattle died in great numbers, and the tsetse fly which had previously fed on them, seeking alternative hosts, began to prey on man and infect them with sleeping sickness. A second effect of the epidemic was bush extension. Foliage, which had previously been controlled by game, now stretched across their old grazing grounds and provided fresh breeding places for fly. Rinderpest also decimated the cattle herds of the pastoral people of East Africa who due to the resulting malnutrition became more susceptible to disease.

The immediate consequences of the final breaching of the old African seclusion was epidemiological disaster. We shall never know how many died from disease during the four decades which followed the European conquest,* but some idea of the loss emerges from figures published admittedly from two particularly unhealthy regions. The inhabitants of the Belgian Congo before 1880 were estimated to number about 40 million; by 1910 the figure had dropped to 15.5 million, and was 9.25 million in 1933. The record from French West Africa is still more shattering: it states that the population of one area was 20 million in 1911; by 1921 it was reduced to 7.5 million and was down to 2.5 million in 1931. By 1936, however, the figure was rising and had reached nearly 3.5 million.

Certainly the years between 1885 and 1930 mark the most unhealthy period of African history, and it is little comfort to acknowledge that the Africans at least fared better than the Polynesians, Melanesians, Australian aborigenes and Amerindians from the white intrusion into the wet tropics; these people, having been denied the Africans' earlier fleeting contact with outside infectious diseases, were almost completely unprotected against imported germs. Nor do we gain much relief by appreciating that eventually Africa had to become part of the outside world with all the consequences of meeting new diseases, and that its conquest by Europe only hastened the inevitable.

The European powers somewhat belatedly recognised their responsibility for indirectly spreading disease through Africa, but once this was appreciated they reacted strongly

* Estimates on the population of Middle Africa before the conquest are notoriously unreliable, varying from 28 million to 180 million (the latter, H.M. Stanley's guess). Probably the figure stood midway between these extremes, at about 100 million.

in an attempt to improve the situation. The elimination of malaria was seen as the first priority. Fortunately a group of men of scientific genius appeared who within sixty years reversed the trend of African morbidity and mortality. Today the population of Africa has risen to over four hundred million, and its peoples are more active physically and mentally than ever before. Much of the credit for this achievement must go to a physician working in China who, during 1879, suspected that some tropical diseases were spread by biting insects, and he went on to prove this. His observations provided scientists with the opportunity of ridding the world of the tyranny of malaria and other tropical dieases and he was to become renowned as 'the father of tropical medicine'.

6

The Father of Tropical Medicine

QUININE MIGHT CURE malaria, but the disease would never be eradicated until the organism which caused it had been identified, its life cycle elucidated, and the method of transmission to man discerned. The first scientific clue to these problems was provided by a young doctor, Patrick Manson, when he was working in a southern Chinese port. Manson had been named after his maternal grandfather, Patrick Baillie, temporarily renowned as surgeon in HMS *Undaunted* when it carried Napoleon to Elba.

Of Orcadian stock, Manson was born in 1844. When only a boy he started work as an apprentice to an iron worker, but strained his back while lifting heavy machinery and decided that manual labour was not for him. Instead he decided to study medicine and graduated at Aberdeen at the age of twenty.

Some years later he accepted an appointment to the Chinese Imperial Maritime Customs, and was posted to a small station in Formosa. Manson was a quiet, kindly man, and he quickly made friends among the Chinese on the island. This association was, however, frowned upon by the authorities and early in 1871 the twenty-seven-year-old doctor was discretely transferred to Amoy on the mainland. Amoy was one of the treaty ports opened to European trade at the end of the Opium Wars; it housed over a quarter of a million Chinese and some hundred and fifty white ex-patriate traders, officials and missionaries. In Amoy Manson found himself in charge of two hospitals. One served white seamen, the other was a missionary establishment which catered for Chinese patients.

Already Manson was intrigued by the strange diseases he

encountered in China, and at Amoy he was particularly struck by the high incidence of elephantiasis among his patients. It was a grossly deforming disease, producing remarkable enlargement of the legs and male genital organs. The scrotum might grow to weigh anything up to twenty kilograms, and it was common to see those unfortunates so afflicted pushing their genitalia in front of them in a barrow. One famous scrotum measured three metres in circumference.

The cause of elephantiasis was unknown, although the Chinese in Amoy were convinced that it was caused by 'a certain dragon', and they attempted to drive away the monster with parades, sacrifices, and letting-off fire crackers. Manson decided that at least surgical removal of enlarged scrotums was practical, and he proceeded to gain great credit among the people in Amoy by conducting thirty successful excisions of the embarrasing deformity. But he was far more interested in the cause of the disease than in its cosmetic relief, and after earnest study he concluded that the swellings must be due to some agent blocking the lymph channels which drain the lower parts of the body, and he determined to find out how this occurred. His research was sadly hindered by the intense repugnance of the Chinese for post-mortem examinations and his investigations nearly ended in tragedy after he bribed a recently widowed woman to allow him to conduct an autopsy on the body of her late afflicted husband; while the post-mortem examination was in progress, a mob rioted outside the house, and Manson had to flee for his life.

He took himself off on leave to Europe in 1874, at a time when exciting progress was taking place in developing medical science. Important advances were being made in France and Germany, and they culminated in the formulation of the germ theory of disease.

For many years European belief accepted that everything in the world was made up from four elements, earth, air, fire and water, and that good health depended on keeping these four elements in judicious balance within the body. It was presumed that disease occurred when these humours became 'alienated', and treatment was then directed at driving out the offending humour through bleeding, purging, inducing salivation with mercury (usually compounded with chalk), and sweating following the administration of guaiacum. Recent improvements in the microscope, however, had made possible the recognition of a large variety of harmful primitive organisms which went under several generic names – germs, microbes, bacteria. These belonged to the plant family and were found to be widely distributed, even in the air. They appeared in various forms: some were minute spheres and these were called cocci; rod-shaped germs were known as bacilli, and spiral filaments termed spirilla or spirochaetes.

During 1868 Louis Pasteur isolated a bacillus which he proved caused disease in silk worms and five years later, just before Manson's return to England, Robert Koch elucidated the life cycle of the anthrax bacillus which was responsible for illnesses in both men and animals. These were but the beginning of remarkable advances. An increasing number of pathogenic germs were identified during the succeeding years, including those which caused tuberculosis and cholera. The new science of bacteriology had been born.

This represented a revolution in medical thought. It had become clear that very small living things, endowed with pathogenic qualities, were responsible for the production of many human diseases. But Manson, while noting these revelations, was only concerned with the problem of elephantiasis, and he attempted to gather all the information about it that could be found. Some quickly turned up in the reading room of the British Museum, at the time much frequented by Karl Marx. To begin with Manson came across a French reference to small snake-like worms which had been found in the scrotal sac of a patient suffering from elephantiasis. The organisms were far larger than the

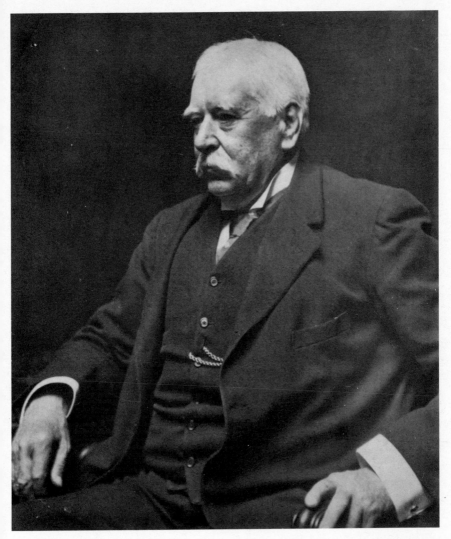

1 Patrick Manson (1844–1922) who first demonstrated the transmission of a
tropical disease by a biting insect. He subsequently became known as 'the
Father of Tropical Medicine'

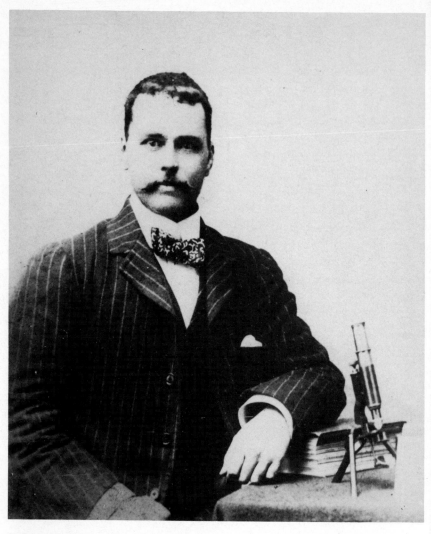

2 Ronald Ross (1857–1932) – the discoverer of the mosquito transmission of malaria

germs described by Pasteur and Koch. Then Manson learned that Timothy Lewis, working in India four years earlier, had seen the same parasites in the urine of a Hindu patient, and subsequently found their minute offspring (larvae) in human blood. Working in Brazil, a researcher named Wucherer described the embryos a little earlier, but his discovery aroused little attention at the time. Subsequently Bancroft, an Australian worker, identified the adult forms of the blood parasites in human lymph tissue, and because of their filamentous shape named them filaria. Manson received no eponymous honour for his work on filariasis, the parasites being alternatively known as *Filaria bancrofti* or *Wucheraria bancrofti*, thus recognising the other two claimants for distinction. The mature female worm was thread-like and fully ninety millimetres in length; the male was thicker but only half as long. Since the embryo forms seen in human blood were microscopic in size they were known as *microfilaria*, or *filaria sanquinis hominis*, that is filaria in human blood.

When Manson returned to Amoy at the end of his leave, he took back several new acquisitions, including a bride, a new microscope, all the available information about elephantiasis, and a determination to fill in the gaps of knowledge about the disease. Almost at once he obtained some interesting results; examination of a random selection of his patients revealed that eleven per cent of them had microfilariae in their blood, and that the incidence was notably higher in those suffering from elephantiasis. By chance he arranged for his two assistants to examine these blood films in alternate twelve-hour shifts, one man employed by day, the other by night. The night worker appeared to be far the more adept at recognising the organisms until Manson discovered the real reason for the discrepancy. He realised that many more microfilariae appeared in the peripheral blood of his patients at night than in the day time.

It was a chance observation but one which was to father

the birth of a new discipline, the practice of tropical medicine. For some time Manson puzzled over this 'periodicity' in the appearance of microfilaria in the host's peripheral blood. Only gradually did he come to appreciate its significance. The 'tide' of microfilaria in the superficial blood stream appeared at exactly the time when his patients were most likely to be bitten by mosquitoes (or possibly other insects) which were searching for blood feeds after sunset. It followed that these insects *might* therefore be the carriers of the disease which by now was known as filariasis.

This appreciation was revolutionary since few people had thought deeply about the possible transmission of disease by insects. Manson reported his findings and speculations to an eminent London entomologist, Spencer Cobbold, in a letter dated 20 June 1879, and Cobbold duly communicated the phenomenon of filarial periodicity to his colleagues. The majority scoffed at Manson's findings and one enquired sarcastically as to whether the tiny organisms carried watches?

But Manson continued the research which was to establish his theory of insect transmission. He calculated that a single patient might carry anything up to ten million filarial embryos in his blood, and he reasoned that if all these microfilariae developed into adult forms, the sheer weight of numbers would destroy their host as well as themselves. It followed, Manson suggested, that if they were to survive, these embryonic forms had to escape in some manner to the outside world. He accepted that a small proportion might be voided in the patient's urine or even in tears, but he conceived that the most likely way they could break loose from their host would be through the medium of biting insects which preyed on human beings and repeatedly extracted their blood. He further suggested that these insects then 'nursed' the embryos they had ingested until the microfilariae were sufficiently mature to reinfect human hosts.

It seemed to him that the secondary host of filariasis

might be one of several biting insects. He dismissed the possibility of bugs, lice, and fleas being responsible since they were found in temperate climates where filariasis did not occur. He considered sand flies as a possible vector, only to dismiss them since they were uncommon in Amoy. This left the prevalent *culex* mosquitoes as the most likely insect host. He knew little about them, and it was typical of the time that when he asked the curator of the Natural History Museum in London to send him a book about mosquitoes, Manson was informed that no such work existed but a book on cockroaches had been despatched to Amoy instead. Despite this setback, Manson determined to test his mosquito theory and he began breeding *culex* mosquitoes in captivity so that he would be certain they were free from filarial infection.

In a vital experiment Manson next fed the 'clean' mosquitoes on his servant Huito whom he knew to be suffering from filariasis. Subsequent dissection of the mosquitoes showed that their stomachs were filled with microfilariae, and further examinations indicated that after a day or two the larvae made their way through the insects' stomach wall to their chest muscles where the embryos underwent further development. Evidently the larvae had matured within the insect's body after two to three weeks and, as Manson put it, were 'on the road to a new human host'. Manson had thus in 1878 confirmed that each embryo in the human blood, after being ingested by the mosquito, was 'nursed' within its body until it could be transmitted back to one of its destined definitive human hosts.

Manson was essentially a reticent man and at the time merely noted that he had 'stumbled on an important point'; he had in fact set tropical medicine on a new and unexpected course, for his experiments proved that at least one disease in the tropics was transmitted by a biting insect and that some human parasites might require two hosts to complete their life cycles. It followed that other diseases too, might be carried by blood-sucking insects which were so common in sub-Saharan Africa. But he was unable fully to understand the phenomenon of filarial periodicity which had uncovered his vital clue, and even today it remains something of a mystery. One researcher suggested that female filariae discharged a new generation of embryos every twenty-four hours, and that each swarm died before the following generation appeared in the blood. Manson, however, effectively demolished this theory when he autopsied a man suffering from elephantiasis who had swallowed a lethal dose of prussic acid. The examination showed that during daylight hours the microfilariae disappeared from the blood vessels of the skin and lodged in those of the lungs and other internal organs. But this observation did not clear up the mechanism of periodicity. All we can be certain about the phenomenon is that it is somehow associated with man's sleeping habits. For people like night watchmen, who sleep by day, harbour the embryos in their superficial blood only during daylight hours, and regular periodicity lapses in air crews who frequently fly at night and sleep during daylight.

Clearly, the appearance of the embryos in available human blood at a time when mosquitoes are foraging, provided filariae with an important survival value, to which the species had gratefully adapted. Yet, although Manson realised that man infected the mosquitoes when the insects fed, he did not appreciate that the mosquitoes in turn infected other men when biting. For he had failed to follow the complete development of the embryos within the mosquito and it was left to later researchers to discover that the larvae eventually entered the sheath of the insect's proboscis (the tube used by biting insects to draw the blood) where they were poised ready to slide into the flesh of the new host during the insect's next act of feeding. Instead, Manson postulated that the life span of mosquitoes was short, and that they deposited their eggs in water shortly before death. The infection was then, according to his theory, transmitted to another human host in the contaminated drinking water.

In Africa filariasis is most common in coastal regions. There, up to sixty per cent of the inhabitants may be affected but they rarely show the gross signs of 'lymph dropsy' which is so common in the Far East. The Africans have clearly developed some degree of immunity to infection, and it is the newcomers who are most at risk from the disease.

Today the adoption of anti-mosquito measures has greatly reduced the incidence of filariasis in the sub-continent, and a drug, diethyl carbamine, now makes possible a complete cure of the disease provided it is given early in its course. Surgery continues to offer relief in lymph scrotum, but good cosmetic results are still difficult to obtain when the legs are affected.

After completing his work on filariasis, Manson moved to Hong Kong and engaged there in so lucrative a practice that he was able to retire to Scotland at the age of forty-six. But his retirement was shortlived; devaluation of his Chinese stock forced him back to work. It was disappointing for Manson but fortunate for Africa. Practising in London from rooms in Queen Anne Street, Manson soon became an oracle for anyone who passed through Britain suffering from tropical diseases. He was the inspiration, too, of the many advances in tropical medicine made during the next thirty years, and it became customary for doctors on leave from British dependencies to seek him out for advice about their local medical problems.

Manson was a stimulating teacher and the lectures he presently delivered in London were always well attended. He constantly sought official support for his policy of teaching his subject to doctors going out to tropical countries and in Joseph Chamberlain, the Secretary of State for the Colonies, he found a vigorous ally. Together the two men pleaded with the General Medical Council in Britain to include diseases of warm climates in the medical students' curriculum, and when the council declined, Chamberlain used all his influence in inducing governors of the tropical dependencies to demand proper training for medical men posted overseas.

With Chamberlain's support Manson opened two wards in the Seamen's Hospital at Greenwich in 1899 for patients suffering from diseases contracted in hot climates. These facilities together with Manson's own laboratory formed the nucleus for a teaching hospital dealing with tropical diseases. At about the same time a group of philanthropists in Liverpool decided to set up their own school of tropical medicine. The impetus for this development came from a gathering of medical students at the Royal Southern Hospital in the city, and they were immediately supported by the shipping magnate, Sir Alfred Jones.* Such interest developed that the Liverpool School actually opened a few months before Manson's institution in London, and after 1900 it received an equal measure of government support.

Up to this time each of the British colonies in Africa had been served by their separate diminutive medical services, many of which had been set up on an *ad hoc* basis. But again Chamberlain acted, and in 1902 the services in West Africa were amalgamated. Next year a similar merger brought unity to those in East Africa, and soon afterwards a comprehensive Colonial Medical Service came into being.

It had its defects of course, especially during the early years: one was the fact that most medical officers were single-handed and running large districts, where they found difficulty in keeping a balance between the curative work demanded by their hospitals and the public health exercises required in the district. Then again the Colonial Office mainly recruited male doctors, and as a result far too little attention was given to pediatric work, a particularly important field, nor were African mothers taught to feed

* Sir Alfred rivals another layman, Sir Henry Wellcome, industrialist and friend of H.M. Stanley, in his services to the elimination of tropical disease. It was Sir Henry who founded the famous research institution which for many years bore his name, the Wellcome Bureau of Scientific Research.

and care for their children properly. Yet the medical service served Africa well, and many of the improvements in the future welfare of its people stemmed from the original vision of Patrick Manson and Joseph Chamberlain.

The establishment of a full Colonial Medical Service was in due course followed by the setting up of medical training centres for African staff at Ibadan, Makerere, Salisbury and other centres in the continent, and these eventually developed into fully fledged medical schools and research centres.

Many medical missionaries also benefited from Manson's lectures, for by 1900 it had become abundantly clear to their societies that missionaries had a duty to minister to the Africans' physical health as well as to their spiritual needs. Medical missionaries had already played a devoted part in bringing the benefits of western medicine to the people of Middle Africa. The first known hospital to serve them was opened in Mozambique by mission workers as early as 1518, and by the end of the century the Franciscans were ministering to the sick in Angola. During 1797 the London Missionary Society recruited its first doctor to work in Africa, and in 1840, David Livingstone sailed for the continent. It was he, more than any other man, who brought the infirmity of Africa to the notice of Europe and America, and his appeals for more workers in the field were taken up by several other societies. Missionary service required almost complete self-surrender, and those that went out suffered grievously in their work. The Wesleyan Missionary Society which sent out two hundred and twenty-five men to West Africa between 1835 and 1907 lost sixty-five of them in the field, while more than half the men serving Africa with the Baptist Missionary Society perished during the decade following 1878.

Many medical missionaries in Africa believed that their patients should make at least a token payment for their treatment; at the end of the nineteenth century, Albert Cook, a pioneer in Uganda, drew up a scale of fees for those attending his clinics in Kampala, though admittedly it varied according to the patient's means rather than to the expense incurred by the Society. An African outpatient would normally be charged five cents (about one penny) but the fee was doubled if he was wearing a European coat. African inpatients were treated free unless admitted for venereal disease. Chiefs and Indians paid about a shilling for a consultation, Europeans and Goanese three times as much.

The medical missionary phase is still very much alive in sub-Saharan Africa, but the old Colonial Medical Service withdrew from the continent after the dependencies gained their independence. Yet the final flowering of the service – the medical school phase – was perhaps its most significant. For greater emphasis was then placed on the training of African doctors and the establishment of medical schools whose teaching was adapted to local circumstances rather than those of western medicine. More interest too, was taken in determining the geographical pattern of disease. This was found to be related to the varying cultural life among different African communities, and in particular to the type of food eaten, but other environmental factors were hardly less important. The surveys stumbled across new diseases like Burkitt's tumour which turned out to have an important bearing on the cause of some forms of cancer, while fibrotic changes in the heart muscle were also recognised which appeared to be related to some immunological response by Africans to malarial infection. All these advances ultimately stemmed from Manson's pioneer labours. Manson's work brought him fame, scientific respect, and a knighthood, but it also engendered professional jealousy and made him enemies. They included officers of the Royal Army Medical Corps who considered that the main school for tropical medicine should have been based on the already famous military hospital at Netley. More serious still was the antagonism which developed between Manson and the equally influential Director of the Natural History Museum in London, Sir Ray Lankester. Lankester was an overbear-

ing man and a formidable antagonist; he even overawed a
governor of Uganda when visiting that infant colony, and
set him grumbling that Sir Ray was 'big and bulky and can be
very rude at times'.

Lankester enjoyed tremendous prestige among the
British public of his day following his introduction to them
of what is now called 'popular science'. Essentially a zoo-
logist who had a flair for writing on his subject in an easy,
comprehensible style, he felt very strongly that the new
science of tropical medicine initiated by Manson must be the
province of biologists rather than of doctors, who, Sir Ray
said, should devote their energies to curing diseases instead
of attempting to find out what caused them. And he was
forever putting this viewpoint forward.

Perhaps because he resented Manson's position at the
Colonial Office and his influence on Joseph Chamberlain,
Lankester went out of his way to denigrate Manson's research, and constantly used his position to hamper the work
of Sir Patrick's protégés. Manson would, however, presently
play a vital part in the elucidation of the life cycle of the
malaria parasite, but he was also to alter world history in
another, quite unanticipated way. When practising in Hong
Kong, Manson founded the nucleus of its present school of
medicine, where one of his most promising pupils was a Dr
Sun Yat-Sen. In 1896 Sun took part in an abortive rising
against the Manchus in China, and, after its failure, fled to
London. On 11th October, Sun was kidnapped by hirelings
of the Chinese embassy while strolling down Devonshire
Street. He was then incarcerated in one of the cellars of the
Chinese legation in Portland Place until he could be transferred secretly to China for trial and, presumably, execu-
tion. Sun, however, managed to smuggle a written message
to Manson when an obliging English servant agreed to carry
it out in a coal scuttle. The appeal for help was duly delivered and Manson together with a colleague, Sir James
Cantlie, mounted guard outside the embassy until a plea
they had sent to the Foreign Office resulted in Sun's release.

Their protégé presently returned to China to lead the revolution which brought down the Manchu dynasty and began the modernisation of the world's largest nation.

While Manson was investigating the etiology of elephantiasis in Amoy, a Frenchman, Alphonse Laveran, was hard at work studying the blood of patients suffering from malaria. He was in his early thirties at the time and had qualified in medicine at Strasbourg. Afterwards Laveran served in the Franco-Prussian war, surviving both the battle of Gravelotte and the siege of Metz. With the coming of peace in 1871, he was posted to Algeria and there began using his primitive microscope to examine the pigmented red blood cells which had already been reported in malarial patients. There are many million red corpuscles in the human body. Most of them are circulated through its larger blood vessels, but a small proportion are at any one time passing through a superficial network of vessels in the skin. It is in these that the blood corpuscles are available as food to foraging insects. On 6th November 1880 he watched entranced as several whip-like filaments or flagella suddenly extruded from one of the affected cells. Laveran appreciated that the 'pigmented bodies' within the cells from which these filaments had originated must therefore be living organisms, and ones which, moreover, might be responsible for malarial fever. Time proved Laveran correct on both counts. The causal organism of malaria had at last been identified. The parasite was presently named 'plasmodium', although strictly the organisms are protozoa. Subsequent work showed that four different species of *Plasmodium* infected man with malaria, each one producing different clinical effects. The most benign form of the disease causes periodic chills and fever but is rarely fatal. Malignant malaria, the killer disease, is caused by the species named *Plasmodium falciparum*.

Other workers quickly confirmed the phenomenon of ex-flagellation in malaria parasites, which occurs about ten minutes after the blood has been drawn, but dispute arose over its significance. Thus some authorities decided that ex-flagellation represented the 'death agony' of the parasite. Laveran disagreed. The flagella, he insisted, were extrusions from a male parasite, and, like sperms, escaped so that they might fertilise female forms of the same parasite. Laveran also suggested that the pigment in the blood parasites represented broken down, 'excrematous' haemoglobin on which the parasites had fed.

Laveran's work represented an enormous step forward in the understanding of malaria. Subsequent experiments by Italian workers demonstrated that the responsible parasite underwent not only the sexual reproductive cycle that Laveran had formulated, but also an asexual form of multiplication by simple division in human blood. Manson's work had already provided a clue to the manner in which Laveran's 'sperms' might escape from man's blood stream, by demonstrating that filaria parasites changed their host when sucked up by a biting insect. If the insect transmitter of malarial parasites could be identified then the other pieces in the puzzle of the malaria life-cycle eventually would fall into their places. It was at this point of time that a young doctor serving in the Indian Medical Service paid an afternoon call on Sir Patrick Manson in his consulting rooms at Queen Anne Street. His name was Ronald Ross. Cynics would later describe him as Manson's greatest discovery.

7

Malaria –
'O million-murdering Death'

POET, MATHEMATICIAN, NOVELIST, artist, musician and
brilliant scientist, Ronald Ross was all these during his
career, and the wearer too of more chips on his shoulder
than almost any other world-famous man. He was born in
the foot-hills of the Himalayas within a few days of the
outbreak of the Indian Mutiny in 1857, the son of a Brig-
adier-General of the Indian Army, who is best remembered
now for his formidable appearance and engaging weakness
for watercolour painting. Like so many children of British
parents in the Far East, Ross was sent home to be educated
at the age of eight.

Young Ross had no intention of following in his father's
military footsteps. He wanted to become an artist, but the
General's mind was set on his being a doctor, and he duly
sent his son to St Bartholomew's Hospital in London, where
he qualified in 1881. Ross later recalled that during his time
at 'Barts' he saw the last case of malaria to occur in England.

By the time he graduated Ross's character was already
ambivalent and complex. He was a self-tormented young
man, deeply emotional, over-sensitive to slights and very
conscious that his talents went unappreciated. Always an
attentive student of his own woes, he came to lack any
capacity for allowing bygones be bygones, and as a result he
passed his life in a state of chronic exasperation, the prey to
all kinds of fears and prejudices. But, as his work would
show, he was also possessed by a sort of genius which was,
however, erratically expressed. It was typical of Ross that as
a medical student he should have spent more time com-
posing poetry and devising systems of shorthand than

reading his textbooks. He only scraped through his quali-
fying examinations.

In appearance Ross was a well-built man who held himself
stiffly, and this, together with his close-cropped hair,
occasional brusqueness and upturned moustache gave
strangers a vague impression of a Prussian officer. It was as
though he tried to hide the sensitivity of his nature behind a
screen of hardness.

At his father's insistence young Dr Ross joined the Indian
Medical Service and served without undue distinction for
several years in India and Burma. He had ample spare time;
during it he studied philosophy and wrote an epic drama.

In 1888 Ross returned on long leave to England where
he took a course in microbiology, published a romance
named *The Child of Ocean* (for which he received £17.17.6 in
royalties) and found time to court and marry a Miss Rosa
Bloxham. Back in India, Ross began to take an interest in
the breeding habits of the mosquitoes which infested his
quarters; he devoured Laveran's enormous tome on malaria, and sought in vain to find his parasites in blood slides.
Ross was brash enough to conclude that Laveran's plasmodia did not exist, and was later embarrassed when his
strictures appeared in print.

Ross was in England again on leave with his wife and two
small daughters during 1894, and he decided to make contact with Manson to obtain his opinion on Laveran's discoveries. He called at 21 Queen Anne Street that April.
Manson greeted him cordially and during the rest of his
leave treated Ross, as the young man gratefully noticed,
'with great kindness' and consideration. No two persons
could have been more different, Ross all heat and passion,
Manson a staid father-figure, and yet these men were to
work very closely together, and to form the most remarkable and fruitful partnership in the history of medicine.

Manson was of course fully aware of Laveran's work on
malaria, but he had not actually seen the parasite until 1892.
He had gone on to verify the phenomenon of ex-flagel-

lation, and was particularly impressed by the fact that it did not occur until the blood had been extracted and cooled. He agreed with Laveran that the process was a means of providing a way for the parasites to continue their existence outside the human body, and considered that research should be directed towards discovering the subsequent development and fate of the flagella.

When Ronald Ross called on him and mentioned that he had never seen malaria parasites, Manson at once demonstrated them in the laboratory on the upper story of his house. More visits to Queen Anne Street followed and one day Manson carried his new pupil off to Charing Cross Hospital to demonstrate the curious crescentic shape adopted by some of the parasites in a patient's blood.

Ross presently took his family on holiday to Switzerland and for a time malaria was forgotten. But on his return to England he once again called on Manson, to find him on the point of leaving to visit the Seamen's Hospital at Greenwich. Ross accompanied him on his way and it was while the two men were walking down Oxford Street to catch a bus that Manson suddenly turned to his companion and said 'Do you know, I have formed the theory that mosquitoes carry malaria just as they carry filaria.' This was one of the first enunciations of what came to be known as 'Manson's mosquito hypothesis' and it was publicly announced only a few days later. His thinking erred in one respect; Manson had not yet accepted that the flagella were sexual forms of the parasite or that they developed further in the mosquito after a blood feed; instead he believed that the infected insect then contaminated drinking water with the plasmodium parasites which in turn were swallowed by a new human host. As with filariasis, he had failed to appreciate that the disease germ was passed on to man again when an infected insect bit him.

Manson's hypothesis aroused a good deal of sceptical comment among his colleagues. They nicknamed him 'Mosquito Manson', and would tap their foreheads knowingly as they watched him go by. Manson was unabashed, and would point at them in turn and tap his own forehead with a gesture of despair.

But Ross was immediately impressed by the hypothesis, and he promised Manson to test it when he returned to India, adding that he would work on mosquitoes rather than on human subjects. When Ross presently landed at Bombay on 21st April 1895, he found himself posted to Secunderabad, a desolate station garrisoned by the 19th Madras Infantry. It was there that he began his research into mosquito transmission, and entered into a period of unremitting toil.

Although he now enthusiastically adopted a new role as scientist, Ross never abandoned his other interests. John Masefield, who came to know him well, paid just tribute to this versatility when he praised Ross as a master of mathematics, an inspired composer, an eminent poet, and 'the most gifted and forceful man it has ever been my privilege to know'. Masefield even declared Ross's *In Exile* to be 'by far the most splendid poem in modern times', a verdict with which few people today would agree. But now Ross became inspired by his new interest. He threw himself into the malaria work with such dediction that he could inform Manson 'I feel a kind of religious excitement over it', and that he dissected each mosquito 'with the same passion and care as one would search some vast ruined palace for a little hidden treasure'. Of all the scientists who researched tropical medicine only Ross could have described his investigations in this matter. Fortunately, his regimental duties were few and he was able to work continuously in the shed which served as his laboratory from seven in the morning till nightfall. His efforts were on a heroic scale: he dissected thousands of mosquitoes under highly unsatisfactory conditions; each dissection was meticulous and liable to take up to two hours; each was performed in a stuffy, ill-lit room, so hot that the sweat ran down his face and rusted the precious microscope he had brought out from England. He would not even allow the working of a punkah lest it blew away his flimsy material.

During this difficult time Ross was very conscious that his labours were frowned upon by the authorities. He became increasingly convinced that his superiors were going out of their way to frustrate him, and indeed his research was interrupted several times on some pretext or another, and precisely when he seemed to be on the point of making some advance in his work.

In his highly emotional state Ross came to believe that 'a ring of five' among his senior officers regarded him as a quack and a nuisance, and looked down on him. There were days when his correspondence to Queen Anne Street was hysterical with frustration, but always in the post were letters in reply from Manson, encouraging him in his research, and all filled with sage and tactful advice. Between April 1895 and the February of 1899 Manson wrote him no less than eighty-five long letters while Ross sent back well over a hundred, each of which averaged a thousand words. When he became celebrated, Ross spoke of Manson's correspondence as 'a noble series such as few men have received' and certainly the two men's letters provide a unique insight into their thoughts and value judgements. As the experiments proceeded, Manson's communications became filled with constructive criticism and edged with high expectations. 'Above all,' he advised Ross during June 1895, 'don't give up. Look upon the task as a Holy Grail, and yourself as Sir Galahad.' He repeatedly recommended Ross to 'follow up the flagella' in his investigations, and at all costs avoid being beguiled into initiating other experiments. In the flagella Manson repeated over and over again, lay the vital clue to malarial transmission. 'I beg of you,' he wrote in the April of 1896, 'not to leave hold of the flagellum.' And so it went on; the friendships of scientists can be as generous as their rages.

In addition to liberating a spate of new ideas, Manson's letters kept Ross in touch with events at home. In one of

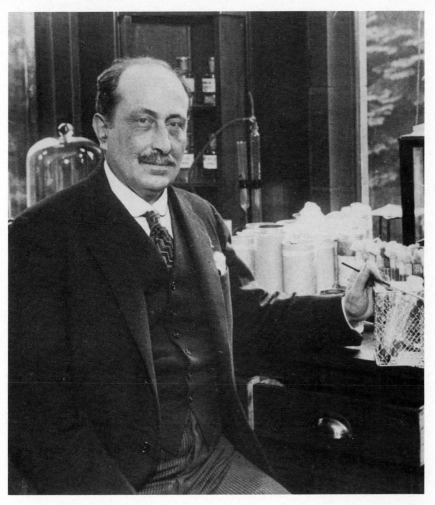

3 Aldo Castellani (1879–1971)–Castellani as a young man demonstrated trypanosomes in the blood of patients suffering from sleeping sickness

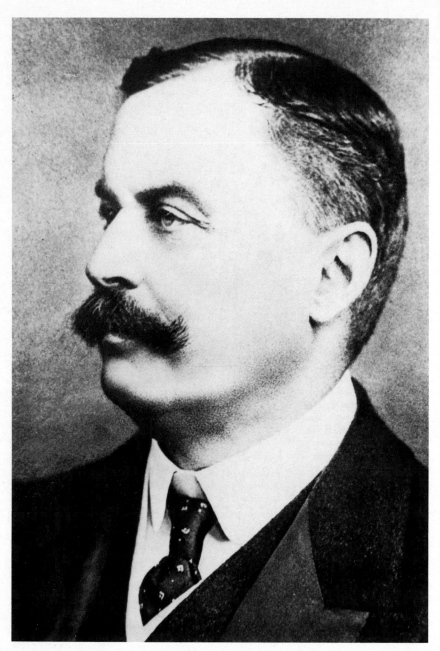

4 David Bruce (1855–1931) – Bruce discovered that nagana was transmitted to animals by tsetse flies in 1895 and eight years later played a large part in identifying the organism responsible for sleeping sickness

them he almost gloated over the death from fever of Prince Henry of Battenberg in Ashanti since it had brought on a 'boom' in malaria. Other letters would indicate some new slant on the disease. Thus he once shrewdly noted that during the sweating stages of malaria, the patient was least able to defend himself against the mosquitoes since he had exposed his skin by throwing off his clothes and was prostrated by his fever.

For some time Ross tried to prove Manson's belief that the female mosquito was shortlived and died soon after depositing eggs in water which, thus contaminated, carried the infection to man. But all Ross's attempts failed to infect volunteers who had been persuaded to drink 'mosquito soup'. This setback made Ross begin a systematic dissection of mosquitoes to discover more about what happened to the flagella after they were ingested. He placed mosquitoes inside a net with his servant, Husein Khan, who suffered from malaria, paying him an anna each time he was bitten. Ross then killed the insects at intervals with chloroform or puff of cigarette smoke, and finally dissected them. Every examination proved inconclusive, for Ross had unfortunately chosen for his experiments a form of mosquito, *Culex fatigans*, which does not 'nurse' human malaria parasites. He daily grew more discouraged.

The turning point came on 16th August 1897 when his insect-catcher brought in a dozen larvae which presently hatched out into mosquitoes that were new to Ross. They had dappled wings and, when resting, tilted themselves head down at an angle of forty-five degrees instead of maintaining the horizontal position of most mosquitoes. These were in fact specimens of *Anopheles stevensi* which is one of the few mosquitoes that transmit malaria to human beings. Ross's luck had turned at last.

The long-suffering Husein Khan was promptly offered to these mosquitoes, and three days later Ross dissected one insect from the batch. In it he was surprised to find a strange dark protuberance projecting from the insect's stomach wall. As he searched additional fields, Ross saw several more of these 'cells' each one of which contained a cluster of black granules that could only be degraded haemoglobin. It was very hot and oppressive on the following day, 20th August. Only two of the new batch of mosquitoes were still alive, but in the one he dissected Ross found the same curious circular cells growing out from its stomach. They were rather larger than in the previous specimen and they too contained pigmented granules. Ross now fully appreciated the fundamental importance of their presence. The tell-tale pigment indicated that they were derived from malaria parasites and, since the cells had grown during the past twenty-four hours, they were clearly developed forms. As Manson wrote to him later 'You have to thank the plasmodium [malaria parasite] that it is fool enough to carry its pigment dung along with it into the mosquito's tissue. Otherwise I suppose you would never have spotted him.'

After this second revelation, Ross went wearily home to tea, and presently fell asleep. He snapped awake a little later with all his lingering doubts dispelled, certain now that he stood on the brink of a monumental discovery.

He knew that only one of his dapple-winged mosquitoes still remained alive and Ross spent a restless night, concerned lest it die before he could examine it. Next morning, trembling with excitement, Ross killed the last of the mosquitoes. In its stomach he saw the same round bodies and again they had increased in size. Two vital facts had now been demonstrated: the anopheline mosquito was clearly one which carried malaria, and the parasites lived and underwent development in the wall of the insect's stomach. Ross, being Ross, poured out his triumph in poetry.

> This day designing God
> Hath put into my hand
> A wondrous thing. And God
> Be praised. At his command,
> I have found thy secret deeds
> O million-murdering Death.

> I know that this little thing
> A million men will save –
> Oh death where is thy sting?
> Thy victory oh grave?

Ross immediately informed his wife of his success and every year afterwards celebrated the anniversary as 'Mosquito Day'. On the 22nd August he reported his findings to Manson and announced with confidence that within two or three weeks he would have demonstrated the entire life cycle of the malaria parasite.

While continuing to work on the dapple-winged mosquitoes, Ross took time off to despatch a report of his discovery for publication in the British Medical Association's Journal, and officially notified the Director General of the Indian Medical Service of his results. He was justified in sounding a note of triumph in these reports; in many ways his achievement was even more significant than Manson's recognition of the mosquito transmission of filariasis. For Manson had stumbled on something in the way Columbus had done when he found America while searching for the Indies. Ross on the other hand had deliberately sought something already predicted – and found it.

It was at this high moment of Ross's career that a heavy blow fell. He received orders to proceed immediately to Bombay for military duty. From Bombay he was posted to Kherwara, which, he afterwards insisted, was used as a punishment station for officers in disgrace. It was free from malaria, so all research ceased. Ross languished for four months in Kherwara which he variously described as 'the unhealthiest hole in India', 'a convict settlement', and the place where he had been more unhappy than ever before. His posting was all the more galling because, if we are to believe Ross who was always inclined to exaggerate his impositions, it was designed to replace an officer who had been given leave to train race horses. His anger was somewhat allayed when his article appeared in the *British Medical Journal*, but the elation was short-lived: Italian workers, protesting that they had never seen Ross's report, presently repeated his work and 'pirated' from him the honour due to the discoverer of malaria transmission.

Thanks to Manson's influence Ross was transferred from Kherwara to Calcutta at the beginning of 1898. Yet even now the authorities showed scant interest in his completing the malaria work on which he was now so brilliantly embarked. It is true that they provided him with a qualified assistant, but he turned out to be 'cold', even 'sceptical' of Ross's results. In any case there were very few anopheles available for dissection in Calcutta, and Ross's Indian patients were unco-operative about providing him with specimens of their blood. So still the vital clue continued to elude him as to how the developing malaria parasites within the mosquito re-infected man.

Manson came to the rescue again with advice for Ross to work on bird malaria, whose parasites were similar to those affecting human beings. His counsel struck a receptive chord: Ross recalled having recently seen a paper by a Dr MacCallum in which he noted ex-flagellation of the malarial parasites in crows. MacCallum also noted that the flagella penetrated and fertilised the female sexual forms of the malaria parasite.

So on St Patrick's Day 1898, Ross began to feed *culex* mosquitoes on crows, weaver birds, pigeons, larks and sparrows, which the insects bite in parts unprotected by feathers, such as the area round the eye. He soon noted that bodies similar to those seen in anopheles developed in the stomach walls of these insects after an avian blood meal. Ross watched their progress in successive mosquitoes – and saw that the cysts eventually burst, releasing numerous rod-like organisms which made their way to the insects' salivary glands. This result was wholly unexpected. Ross by then was 'nearly blinded with exhaustion' but he appreciated that he now possessed evidence that the mosquito transmitted malaria to the birds by biting, and presumably did the same to man. It was a second breakthrough. Manson on learning of it, delightedly notified Ross's achievement to a medical meeting on 24th July 1898.

But there still remained a flaw in Ross's evidence. He had suggested but failed to demonstrate that malaria transmission in humans occurred in the same way as in birds. It was all the more frustrating, when it only required a single demonstration of infecting man from an anopheline mosquito to solve the whole complicated problem, that at this crucial moment Ross was posted to Assam with orders to work on a totally different disease, Kala Azar, in preference to malaria.

But already Italian workers had completed Ross's task by applying to human malaria the principles he had worked out in birds. Late in July 1898 Professor B. Grassi and his colleagues fed infected anopheline mosquitoes on a volunteer named Adele Sola who was free from malaria. Sola, in due time, went down with a typical attack of fever. The transmission of malaria was thus practically demonstrated, and the total eradication of the disease throughout the tropics was now within reach.

Ross never forgave the Italian workers for what he termed their 'Roman brigandage'. Their task, he said, had merely been to apply his experiments 'when I was prevented by interruptions from doing so, [and] which involved work of no difficulty whatsoever'. He loudly accused these 'scientific kleptomaniacs' of inaccuracy in their work and even of falsifying their results. Grassi, he complained, was a charlatan as well as a thief, while of the Italian workers in general he sneered confusedly that 'great would have been their honour – if their honour had been greater'. His criticism was not entirely justified. Grassi may have been guided in his experiments by Ross's discoveries, but he soon went far further than his British colleague in unravelling the mysteries of the malaria cycle. For in extended experiments the Italian workers identified the four different forms of human malaria parasites, and confirmed the role of quinine in suppressing their asexual (though not their sexual) form of multification.

These advances increased Ross's indignation, as did the provision by Manson of additional proof of malaria transmission of the disease in two practical experiments. He first obtained infected mosquitoes from Grassi in Rome and fed them on his son and another volunteer. Both men went down with malaria a few days later. Then Manson arranged for two colleagues, G.C. Low and L.W. Sambon, to live for three months in the Campagna outside Rome, screened during the night in a mosquito-proofed hut. The experiment aroused great interest, and many eminent men including the King of Italy came to see them. Both Low and Sambon remained free from fever, although the peasants in the area suffered severely from it. There could now be no doubt about the sinister role played by the anopheline mosquito in the transmission of malaria.

In parenthesis it seems fitting that this vital experiment should have been carried out in the Campagna which at the height of the Roman power had been an enormous market garden supplying the nearby city. Then, during the first century BC, the Campagna had become infested with malaria-carrying mosquitoes, and both the live birth-rate and vitality of the Roman citizens began to decline. Within four centuries the Romans had lost their taste for war and were slipping into decadence. Historians now account malaria one of the prime causes of the fall of the Roman Empire.

Frustrated and embittered by the obstructive tactics of his superiors, distressed that the 'great passion' for his work on malaria had 'died' within him, Ross retired from the Indian Medical Service in 1899. He then took a badly paid teaching post at the new Liverpool School of Tropical Medicine, but after a bout of more injustice-collecting resigned in order to resume the study of his earlier love, mathematics. Yet, presently conscience pricked him and he threw himself with something of his old dedication into pioneering methods of sanitary control of mosquito breeding places in tropical

Africa. He opened the campaign against the anopheline
enemy at Freetown and subsequently visited Gambia, Nigeria, Ghana and Egypt to advise on, and sometimes angrily
dictate, methods of malaria control. This work he afterwards maintained was far more significant than his experiments in India, and he once declaimed that 'Great is
sanitation – the greatest work, except discovery, I think, that
a man can do.' The subject even inspired a poem, which is
fairly typical of Ross's style:

> We cry, God, make us kings,
>   Poets or prophets here.
> The scornful answer rings,
>   'First be my scavenger'.

The world recognition which he craved came to Ross in
the end. He received the Nobel Prize and was knighted in
1911. Yet this man, so rich and powerful spiritually, so
impoverished by his fear of being patronised, appears to
have become unbalanced by his triumphs. He became even
more embittered and intolerant of his colleagues, forever
contemplating the deceits of scientific glory with sad
despair. He presently even turned on Manson, conceiving
that he had taken more than his fair share of the credit for
proving mosquito transmission, and he sneered that his old
mentor's laboratory techniques were so prejudiced by his
'shaky hands' that he had failed to be a 'very expert investi-
gator'. Ross even demanded the return of the 'mosquito'
letters he had written to Manson, which by now had become
of immense historical value, and Manson meekly sent them
back.* But perhaps what most brings out Ross's confused
feelings for his former patron appears in his private
memoirs where he wrote: 'It is of course the common duty
of all medical men to help each other when necessary, and
when I received the Nobel Prize in 1902 I did not feel called
upon to divide it with Manson, even if I had thought it

* Ross sold his archives later to Lady Houston for £2,000. She subsequently presented them to the Ross Institute.

proper to do so at all.' Relations between the two men remained strained until Manson's death.

In due course Ross went into private practice in London. He served with distinction in the Army Medical Corps during the Great War and twice survived being torpedoed. His elder son was killed during the retreat from Mons; this tragedy, followed by the deaths of his wife and daughter, saddened Ross's declining years and he dropped into limbo, providing only rare glimpses of himself for future historians to describe. During 1932 he published a plodding autobiography filled with interminable details about the quarrels with his Italian colleagues and the moghuls of the Indian Medical Service. Unarguably one of mankind's greatest benefactors, Ronald Ross, soon afterwards died at the Ross Institute and Hospital for Tropical Diseases which had been founded in his honour six years earlier.

Ross and his Italian rivals had in fact failed to demonstrate every detail of the malaria parasite's life cycle. Two enigmas remained to be explained. To begin with it was not clear why a patient sometimes relapsed from malaria long after leaving the tropics and following apparent cure. The second mystery concerned the fact that when parasites were injected into a subject by a mosquito they disappeared from the peripheral blood within half an hour, and only returned to it a week later; and it was demonstrated that during this week-long latent period the malarial patient could not re-infect a clean mosquito. A suspicion grew that soon after entering the human blood stream, the parasites 'hid' in the host's liver and other internal organs, where they were immune to drug therapy. Shortly before the Second World War experiments on birds showed that these theories were well founded.

During wartime studies conducted by Sir Neil Hamilton Fairley and his colleagues in Queensland on the suppression of malaria attacks by atebrin (work which enabled the Allies to reconquer New Guinea from the Japanese), it was confirmed through transfusion to human volunteers that blood becomes free from parasites soon after an infected mosquito bite. Four years later the postulated 'exo-erythrocytic' forms of the parasite were demonstrated in the liver of a human volunteer. Subsequent experiments showed that one stage of parasite sheltered in the liver for very long periods, and only reappeared in the blood when the human host underwent some form of stress. The demonstration finally explained the delayed attacks of fever which occurred long after patients had left a malarial area.

Later a great deal of research was conducted into the habits of the two thousand seven hundred separate species of mosquitoes that have been identified. It was found that the malaria-carrying mosquitoes are blind in the dark but possess sensors in their two antennae which enable them to seek out their human victims. They make their approach flight along the stream of carbon dioxide exhaled by their prey and calculate their distance to them from the changing concentrations in the air of moisture, warmth and ingredients of human sweat. The latter also provides the mosquitoes with information about the desirability of the prospective victim, some persons being more attractive to biting insects than their more fortunate fellows.

The mosquitoes' feeding processes turned out to be no less marvellous than their tracking techniques. The insect's proboscis consists of six hair-like stylets: two are used for piercing the human skin, two saw the wound open, and the third pair are used to suck out the blood-feed, but only after a minute quantity of saliva has been injected through them into the wound in order to prevent the blood clotting into an indigestible mass in the mosquito's stomach.

But far more than academic success flowed from the recognition of the anopheline mosquito as a vector of malaria and the unravelling of the parasite's life cycle. For thanks to Ross's lead in developing sanitary methods in the field, complete control of malaria could now be contemplated through mounting direct attacks on its mosquito vectors. As long before as 1821 an attempt had been made to drain the swamps round Freetown in Sierra Leone to prevent mosquito breeding, and, less usefully, regular fires had been kindled round their periphery and even a wall, ten metres high and twenty-six kilometres long, was built along the shore line to exclude 'miasma' from the port. Now, ninety years afterwards, screening of houses was instituted in the tropics, while war was declared on larvae in mosquito breeding places. Attempts were made to dry up pools, and if this failed the larvae were suffocated with oil films poured on the water or poisoned with Paris green. In many areas it became an offence to allow the mosquito breeding places to exist on private premises, and the judicial application of fines led eventually to places like Mombasa becoming malaria-free for the first time in history.

The attack on the adult mosquitoes was intensified after the discovery of the residual insecticidal virtues of DDT. This and other long acting insecticides were then applied on a vast scale by spraying a suspension or solution of DDT on the walls of houses where it might remain effective for up to six months. But unfortunately the fecundity of the mosquitoes and their extraordinary adaptability to meet any new threat was underestimated, and as early as 1951 the insects were demonstrating a high resistance to DDT, due either to the selection of strains naturally resistant to the insecticide or by not resting on treated surfaces.

Moreover, DDT turned out to be lethal to forms of animal life other than insects: falcons, sea lions and salmon were among many which showed sensitivity to it, and its application became highly unpopular among a conservation-conscious public.

Similar insecticides like dieldrin and chlorane were also developed in the laboratory with excellent immediate results, but again selective survival of the more resistant strains of mosquitoes vitiated successes. Recourse to an insecticide naturally occurring in a plant, pryrethrum, showed that it possessed a greater immediate effect, although not so long-acting as the synthetics.

It has been suggested that the eradication of mosquitoes from a malarial region might in the long run be potentially dangerous to its inhabitants. For with time they would inevitably lose their hard-won immunity and the chance re-introduction of infected mosquitoes to their countries would result in devastating epidemics.

It has also been appreciated that it might be useless to banish mosquitoes from human living areas, unless apes and monkeys in neighbouring bushlands were also protected against the insects. These creatures suffer from several types of malaria closely resembling the human forms. It is, however, extremely unlikely that their parasites might fill any ecological niche by infecting man.

Clearly the eradication of malaria by attacking its vector faced all sorts of pitfalls and might even be counter-productive. Today it appears that the development of a malaria vaccine is likely to provide the most promising form of preventing the disease.

More advantages have been drawn from the advances in malarial therapeutics. Quinine served mankind well for many years but its drawbacks – its bitter taste, the deafness it caused, the frequent association with vomiting and the dreaded blackwater fever – were fully appreciated. A search therefore was made for synthetic malaria-cides. First atebrin (also known as mepacrine) was introduced and proved to be a more effective drug than quinine. This was followed in 1960 by the appearance of chloroquine which possessed even greater potency and was free from the side effects of atebrin. It has long remained in use and, because it was so effective and cheap, development of resistance by plasmodia to the drug came to be a tragedy for Africa. Subsequently paludrine was synthesised. It possessed the great advantage of being effective against malaria parasites during their sojourn in the liver, and so prevented relapses of the disease. Quite recently the virtues of daraprim and allied drugs have been widely accepted (though daraprim may occasionally damage the bone marrow), and frequent additions to the armoury of malariologists are now being made. Yet still the nagging fear remains that if effective therapy be provided for all the inhabitants of Black Africa and malaria infection becomes a rarity, it will be at the cost of a massive loss of immunity among its inhabitants, a situation that might in the long term prove disastrous unless, like the eradication of smallpox, it is world wide.

8

The Ravages of Sleeping Sickness

TOWARDS THE END of 1900, two brothers, Albert and Jack Cook, who were pioneer medical missionaries in Uganda, congratulated themselves on the conclusion of three gratifying years' work. They had set up a bush hospital at Mengo, now part of modern Kampala, and it was opened to patients on 22nd February 1897, when Ross was still poring over his microscope in Secunderabad and making excited notes on the phenomenon of ex-flagellation in malaria parasites. From there they reported on the wide varieties of diseases they had encountered in Uganda. 'Fever', most of which was thought to be malarial, had proved their greatest problem, but relapsing fever and syphilis had also been common, as well as septic infections, elephantiasis, liver abscess, guinea worm infestation and yaws. During the first year of work they had admitted one hundred and forty-one patients to hospital; since then the number had steadily increased to over a thousand in 1900.

Suddenly, during 1901, the situation at Mengo dramatically altered: their little hospital was besieged by hordes of patients who were suffering from a virulent disease that was new to Uganda, and for which no effective cure was available. At the same time a nearby government medical officer was gloomily recording that some twenty to thirty thousand Africans were either dead or dying in his district. All those, he noted, who were suffering from the new disease (which the Africans named 'n'tola') were carried away from their villages and abandoned in the forest. Their symptoms were macabre: the dying patients exhibited an extravagant sensitivity to cold and a morbid craving for meat. This led them to set their huts on fire to provide warmth and to eat the bodies of the dead and even parts of their living flesh. Albert Cook later remembered that local chiefs were told to bring in a twig for everyone known to have died. 'On the first day,' he wrote, 'the twigs numbered eleven thousand, and the sad little processions continued several days later. . . .' Before the epidemic subsided an estimated three hundred thousand people had died in Buganda alone and the death toll in the Congo Free State was believed to be half a million.*

The Cooks presently reported that the symptoms of the epidemic were suspiciously like those caused by sleeping sickness in West Africa, and that nearly all the patients harboured microfilaria in their blood: (this last was a significant observation because Manson had lately suggested that sleeping sickness was caused by *filaria perstans*, an organism whose larval forms resembled those causing elephantiasis.) Sleeping sickness had been previously unknown in East Africa, and the Cooks' grave news was promptly transmitted to the Colonial Office in London. It was realised there with alarm that sleeping sickness, which had previously been limited to small endemic foci in West Africa, had now spread across the continent to Lake Victoria. The outbreak presented an immediate challenge to the officials who claimed that their recent annexations in Africa had, for their prime motive, a desire to bring the blessings of civilisation and science to their new subjects. Accordingly Sir Patrick Manson was at once approached for advice; so was Sir Ray Lankester, and the influential Council of the Royal Society.

Between them they arranged for a commission of three medical men to go out to the stricken areas and report on

* By 1880 sleeping sickness had been reported from Senegal, Gambia, Sierra Leone, Ivory Coast, and the Gold Coast. During the next three decades, in a classic example of the extension of tropical infection following the European conquest of Africa, it spread to Nigeria, the Cameroons, Portuguese and Spanish Guinea, French Equatorial Africa, Uganda, the Congo Free State, Tanganyika, Nyasaland, the Rhodesias, Bechuanaland and Mozambique.

the cause of the outbreak. It was an important step in the history of medicine in Africa. For this was the first occasion a European government had despatched a research team to the continent to deal with a medical crisis. Two of the commissioners were protégés of Manson; the third was a disciple of Lankester, and known to be difficult and cantankerous. The search for the cause of sleeping sickness was accordingly bedevilled by the same kind of rivalries which had attended the investigations of malaria transmission.

Sleeping sickness, or trypanosomiasis, had been known in West Africa for many centuries. Its symptoms vary with respect to the rapidity of the course of the disease and to its severity. In West Africa the illness among natives tended to be a chronic one, and several years passed before death occurred. But the Ugandan infection clearly ran a far more rapid course, being fatal within a few weeks or months. Though no-one realised it at the time, the rapidity and severity of sleeping sickness in East Africa was due in part to the absence there of any immunity to the disease among its people.

All cases of sleeping sickness begin with an intermittent fever; this is followed by a swelling of the lymphatic glands, particularly those at the back of the neck. The terminal stage of the disease is characterised by inflammation of the brain which results in increasing lethargy, alteration in behaviour,* mania and death, or to some intercurrent infection after the patient has been reduced to helpless inertia.

An epidemic of sleeping sickness was a dreadful thing for a medical officer to handle. This was the only disease which

---

* Indeed one of the earliest symptoms of sleeping sickness may be behavioural changes like irresponsibility and irritability. A European lady once made an urgent appointment for her daughter with a Parisian specialist in tropical medicine, since the girl had developed a fever and headaches in West Africa. The mother later rang up to cancel the appointment because she wished to go to a local dress show. On this slim evidence the specialist diagnosed sleeping sickness in both the girl and her irresponsible mother, and he was perfectly correct.

could wipe out entire communities. A doctor encountering an outbreak was likely to find huts filled with dying patients, together with those who had become maniacal and had been chained to huge logs lest they attacked the few villagers brave enough to bring them scraps of food. The memory of such an outbreak lingers on in Africa's folk lore. Sixty years after one epidemic a white traveller was advised to move his camp. The spirits of N'tola lived there, it was explained, and might cause the sickness to break out again if they were disturbed.

Within a few years of its sudden appearance beside Lake Victoria, sleeping sickness had spread across Africa between about 12° north and 25° south, that is roughly between a line linking the mouth of the Senegal River with Mogadishu, and the Zambezi to the south. Yet much of this huge area had been free from the disease not long before. Livingstone, for example, during his travels, wrote often about the biting habits of the tsetse flies, and although bitten often never went down with sleeping sickness nor mentioned that any Africans he encountered suffered from it. He sent a specimen of tsetse fly home which he later used as a frontispiece to his book *Missionary Travels*. Unfortunately, the fly's head came off on its way to England and was there reattached to the body upside down which is how it appears in the book.

The sleeping sickness commission sent out hurriedly from Britain was confronted by two main problems: its members had to seek out the cause of the disease; secondly they were required to recommend methods of treatment for the affected population and, if possible, ways of controlling the outbreak. In addition they were to attempt to explain the circumstances which had led to the enormous extension of sleeping sickness.

They had little knowledge to help them; no convincing evidence was available about the cause of the disease, though, as with malaria, plenty of theories existed; nor had any satisfactory treatment for sleeping sickness yet been found. Without much guidance the party set off from London on 1st May 1902.

Although they were unaware of the fact, there already existed certain clues which might have led them to an early solution of their problems. Only a short time before on the west coast of Africa a surgeon named Forde had been consulted by an English master of a steamer plying the Gambia River. He had gone down with fever. The patient's blood showed parasites which were quite unlike those associated with malaria. The organism was an active, spindle-shaped body which was spirally twisted and possessed an attached undulating membrane which allowed it to swim rapidly about in the blood. The patient presently relapsed and was referred to a Dr Everett Dutton. Dutton also observed the unusual parasites and reported them to be trypanosomes similar to ones described in rats during 1877.*

Trypanosomes had also recently come into prominence in Natal thanks to some brilliant work performed by an army doctor named David Bruce. Bruce was a man worth studying. He was born in Melbourne in 1855, two years before Ross, but when he was five his father took him back to Scotland to live at Stirling. At the age of fourteen young Bruce was obliged to work for his living and for three years he laboured in a factory in Edinburgh. By the time he was twenty-one he had accumulated enough money to enter Edinburgh University to study zoology, but presently switched to medicine and qualified during 1881. Bruce then

---

* It is interesting to note that Manson nearly achieved priority in discovering a trypanosome in the blood of a sleeping sickness case. During 1900 he examined a patient from the tropics who suffered from a fever of unknown origin. After a preliminary examination the man left the surgery while Manson settled down to examine his blood – and in it recognised a trypanosome. Manson hurried round to his patient's club to obtain more blood for another slide, but by then his subject had been drinking and was pugnacious. Perhaps he was already suffering from encephalitis. At all events he refused to provide a second sample and Manson had to give up the search.

practised as an assistant at Reigate, and there fell in love with Mary Steele, the daughter of his principal. Bruce promptly decided to join the Army Medical Service where his pay as a captain would enable him to marry, and he was posted almost at once to Malta. His was an ideal marriage; from its beginning his wife served as a devoted assistant acting as both microscopist and secretary, and he afterwards insisted that many of the successes which followed were largely due to her work. She died during 1931, and her husband followed only four days later while a memorial service was being held for her in a nearby church.

In Malta, Bruce found that the troops and civilians there were plagued by prolonged attacks of an obscure fever. Using the laboratory techniques learnt from two German scientists, Koch and Klebs, Bruce was able to isolate the bacterium responsible for the disease, and to introduce preventive methods which were to eliminate Malta fever from the island and neighbouring countries. It was the first indication of Bruce's flair and competence in scientific research.

Back in England Bruce became Assistant Professor in Pathology at Netley, the Army Medical Corps hospital in England, where, during 1889, he met Sir Walter Hely-Hutchinson whom he had known in Malta. Hely-Hutchinson was, presently appointed Governor of Natal, and he insisted on the Bruces coming out to South Africa with him to investigate a veterinary disease there named 'nagana'* which was killing large numbers of cattle and horses in the colony. It was associated by the Africans with the bites of tsetse flies. However it was not known at this time to affect domestic animals or monkeys (with the exception of baboons).

---

* Nagana was the Zulu name for the cattle disease due to trypanosomiasis. It means 'low spirits', and was one of the few Africans words which was quickly assimilated into the English language. Bruce might as easily have used another Zulu word – 'munca' – which means 'sucked out', a good description of the appearance of infected cattle.

Tsetse flies greatly hindered Arab attempts to penetrate Black Africa from across the Sahara by killing their horses and camels, and in doing so prevented the mass conversion of its residents to Islam. More significantly nagana disastrously affected the economy of Middle Africa. Lacking draught animals in many areas because of nagana, the Africans could only hand-plough small plots of land, and the transport of goods was limited to what could be carried as head-loads. In addition, the lack of cattle meant that the diet of most people was short of first-class protein and because they had no manure they were obliged repeatedly to break new ground as the fertility of their gardens declined.

David Livingstone had learned from the Africans of the fly's association with a fatal cattle disease, and was surprised that game appeared to be immune to their bites. As early as 1849 he had emphasised the fly was a 'barrier to the progress' of the continent.

The tsetse fly is a bustling, biting insect which is a little larger than a house fly. At rest it can be recognised by the way its wings fold up like scissors. Livingstone came to the conclusion that the fly injected a venom when biting in the same way as poisonous snakes. He even identified 'a bulb at the root of the proboscis' which contained the poison. His findings were well known to Bruce.

When he arrived in Natal, Bruce accordingly learned all he could from local Africans about the habits of tsetse flies, and set up his camp near the village of Ubombo on top of a hill overlooking a well-recognised fly belt. As his first step, he examined the blood of cattle suffering from nagana and in them found trypanosomes in large numbers. His investigations then followed a pattern which would become standard. He sent a healthy horse down from his hill top to the fly country below. Within a short time it sickened and Bruce demonstrated trypanosomes in its blood. He then repeated the experiment with cattle and dogs and found that they too became infested with trypanosomes. The next step was to demonstrate that it had not been 'miasma' or poisoned pasturage which caused the disease. To do this Bruce brought tsetse flies from the valley to the hill top and fed them there on healthy animals. These too soon showed 'tryps' in their blood, members of a strain which was later named *Trypanosoma brucei* in his honour. Finally Bruce bred 'clean' flies and fed them on game and subsequently on domestic animals. All of the latter went down with nagana. It was a thoroughly convincing demonstration that tsetse flies carried nagana, and that the disease was not due to venom as Livingstone suggested, but caused by animal parasites which are carried by tsetse flies without harm to themselves. Unfortunately no-one applied the results to human beings; no thought was given to the possibility of fly-borne nagana being related to sleeping sickness in man.

We next hear of David Bruce serving with distinction as a surgeon in the garrison of Ladysmith when it was under siege by the Boers, with Mrs Bruce inevitably acting as his theatre sister. Following its relief, Bruce became a member of a committee concerned with the prevention of typhoid and dysentery in the British army in South Africa, and subsequent work led to the development of an anti-tetanus vaccine which saved many lives during the First World War. Bruce returned to England very soon after the departure of the first sleeping sickness commission to Uganda and the almost simultaneous recognition of a trypanosome in the blood of a ship's master in Gambia.

By this time Bruce was a celebrity, and his fame seemed to have accentuated some of the less lovable qualities in his character. His mind became blinkered by all manner of prejudices; he disliked foreigners, Jews, and most particularly anyone who disagreed with him. To these people he was brusque, even rude. Yet he could be thoughtful, kind and even humble. He was naturally committed to the advancement of the Royal Army Medical Corps and was an admirer of Sir Ray Lankester. These influences inevitably made him an opponent of Sir Patrick Manson, especially as Bruce believed that Manson had paid him less than his proper due for his work on nagana, an attitude which stood out in sharp contrast to the indulgence Manson had shown to Ross's success in malaria. Yet it could not be denied that Bruce knew more about trypanosomes than anyone else on earth, and now in 1902 he was impatient for further success and fame.

But Bruce's influence on the work of the sleeping sickness commission still lay in the future when its three members (whom a doctor in Uganda rightly considered to be 'a queer lot') assembled in London. The first to be chosen was George Carmichael Low, one of Manson's protégés, whom he had sent out like a human guinea pig to live in a mosquito-proofed house on the malarial Roman Campagna. Low was now thirty years old, a reliable and intelligent man whom the Royal Society's committee appointed to be chairman of the commission. Unfortunately, Low had done very little work in Africa; he had been selected purely for his skill in parasitology.

Cuthbert Christy, the second member of the commission, was senior to Low in age and experience. He had served in Nigeria for some years, was renowned as a 'field man' and had already been elected a Fellow of the Royal Society. Christy was deeply distressed because he had not been chosen as leader of the expedition, and on this account had several times lost his temper during the passage out to Africa. He finally came to blows with Low on Mombasa railway station when he noticed that the carriage of the train taking them up country was labelled 'Dr Low's party'. As it happened neither Low nor Christy were to play significant parts in the elucidation of the sleeping sickness problem. What success was achieved fell almost by accident to the third and youngest member of the team, Dr Aldo Castellani.

Castellani was only twenty-four when Manson chose him as bacteriologist to the commission, after the original candidate had dropped out. Destined to become as controversial a figure as Bruce, Castellani had graduated as a doctor in Florence and then travelled to London to attend

Manson's lectures in tropical medicine. He became devoted
to his tutor and afterwards recalled 'the admiration and
affection I immediately felt for him. He was lovable, kind-
hearted, courteous and paternal. He was indeed a father to
me.' Castellani unhesitatingly accepted Manson's theory
that sleeping sickness was caused by a type of filaria similar
to the one responsible for elephantiasis, and he set out for
Uganda, intending to prove it. Low too had volunteered for
the hazardous expedition to Lake Victoria in order to show
that his chief's theory was correct. Christy had no such
motive.

After a tiresome journey the commissioners arrived
safely on 8th July at the railhead of Kikuyu. From there they
tramped on foot to Lake Victoria. The little party was
headed by a Goanese cook they had engaged, who being
mounted on a donkey, was taken by the flustered Africans
they met to be the head of the expedition. At the lake the
commissioners split up. Christy took himself off into the
bush to demarcate the distribution of sleeping sickness.
After confirming that this did not coincide with that of
filariasis, he lost his taste for the commission's work and,
according to his colleagues, 'became more interested in
butterflies' and hunting.

Meanwhile the two young men, Low and Castellani, made
their way to Entebbe which at the time was no more than 'a
straggling conglomeration of grass-roofed huts'. There,
without much local co-operation, they supervised the construction of a rough mud building which was to combine the
functions of hospital and laboratory. They then went to
work on Manson's filarial theory.

To their distress they soon discovered that local medical
officers had already discredited the hypothesis by demonstrating that filaria infestation was present in areas free
from sleeping sickness. The disappointed Low decided to
return to England where he had been offered a teaching
post, and Christy followed soon afterwards. Castellani
was not so precipitate. He believed he had discovered

an association of the disease with a streptococcus which repeatedly turned up at post mortems. This was in fact hardly surprising; the sleeping sickness patients had been driven out of their villages like lepers and became covered with suppurating sores due to streptococci.

Castellani, alone now in his hut, became restless and a prey to nerves, probably because he was shunned as a foreigner by most of the Europeans in Entebbe, and particularly by his few medical colleagues in Uganda who, with some reason, believed themselves more capable of solving the sleeping sickness puzzle than this Italian theoretician from London. However, Castellani continued his search for more evidence of a streptococcal cause for sleeping sickness and on 12th November 1902 he drew off some cerebo-spinal fluid (the fluid that surrounds the brain and spinal cord) from one of his patients and searched it for streptococci. Instead, in a classic example of serendipity, he saw 'a fish like parasite darting about in the fluid'. It was a little larger than a blood cell, with an undulating membrane attached to the body which vibrated rapidly and propelled the organism through the blood and tissue fluids. Castellani recognised it as a trypanosome similar to those already reported in rats by Timothy Lewis and in cattle by Bruce. But he had not read the report by Dutton and Forde about a trypanosome in the blood of the ship's captain on the Gambia which had appeared two months earlier. Three days later Castellani found a trypanosome in a second case, and an autopsy later recovered trypanosomes from blood and cerebro-spinal fluid.

Even now Castellani believed these organisms were no more than harmless commensals, lacking any association with sleeping sickness, and as late as the February of 1903, he was still proudly showing off his streptococci to Albert Cook as the causal agent of the disease. He was loth to make a fool of himself by any premature disclosure of his finding trypanosomes in his patients, but he continued to look for them in the cerebro-spinal fluid which he now concentrated by centrifuging (rapid spinning), and by 15th March had found them in six more cases. But still he resisted committing himself by stating that these organisms were in fact responsible for human trypanosomiasis, and clung tenaciously to his streptococcus theory. It was at about this stage of his investigations that Castellani learned that London was sending out a second commission to study the disease, and that it was already on its way. For the committee of the Royal Society, which had organised the first expedition, was concerned by the muddled, inconclusive results which had characterised the first commission's work and at Low's abrupt return. Although desperately short of funds the committee decided it must redeem the situation by sending out a second, reinforcing commission to Entebbe. The leader was to be the formidable David Bruce, who very fortunately did not need to be paid since he was a serving officer of the RAMC. It was purely coincidental that he was also the world's authority on trypanosomes; no word of Castellani's discovery of their association with sleeping sickness had yet leaked out. Bruce presently set off with his wife and a laboratory assistant named Gibbons, together with a small, retiring doctor named David Nabarro. Unfortunately, Nabarro had already unintentionally offended the prickly Bruce for, when the project was first bruited, Nabarro had been chosen as 'head' of the new expedition. He suffered in Bruce's eyes from another defect: he had been chosen for the post by Manson. Nabarro admittedly had quickly agreed to serve under Bruce when the older man was chosen as second member of the commission, but the damage had been done. All the ingredients for a first-class row over the priority of any medical discoveries were thus assembled when Bruce's party arrived at the straggling lake-side village of Entebbe on 16th March 1903.

The week of the second commission's arrival at Entebbe witnessed a remarkable coincidence. On 12th March 1903, Dr C.J. Baker, the government medical officer in the station, found trypanosomes in the blood of an African policeman who displayed symptoms of sleeping sickness. Soon afterwards Baker discovered the parasite in two other patients. Baker took his slides along to Castellani who confirmed the identity of the parasite. Under a bond of secrecy he told Baker that he had recently seen the same parasite in the cerebro-spinal fluid of sleeping sickness patients, but he still maintained that they were no more than contaminants and that streptococci were the organisms responsible for the disease.

But Baker, who was aware of Bruce's work on nagana, was more alert. He suspected that these trypanosomes might also be carried by tsetse fly and he set about collecting specimens of the fly in the area. On the day Bruce arrived, Baker showed him the small collection of tsetse he had found. The demonstration must have given Bruce a great deal to think about.

Bruce was in for a second surprise two days later. On 18th March he had a confidential talk with Castellani. After speaking for some time about his attempts to incriminate a streptococcus as the cause of sleeping sickness, Castellani confided to Bruce that he had seen trypanosomes in the blood and cerebro-spinal fluid of several of his patients who had gone down with the disease. But he did this only after laying down certain conditions. Castellani insisted that he be allowed to remain in Entebbe for a few more weeks so that he might continue his work on his streptococcal theory, that any findings he made must be published over his own name, and that nothing about the trypanosome be told to Nabarro. Surprisingly, Bruce agreed to all these terms.

Castellani's insistence on these conditions was unprofessional, and Bruce is open to criticism for accepting them. At all events, while Nabarro was banished for three weeks from the laboratory to make clinical assessments of the sleeping sickness patients, Castellani demonstrated to Bruce his techniques of lumbar puncture (the minor operation of 'tapping' cerebro-spinal fluid by inserting a long needle in the spinal canal) and of centrifuging the cerebro-spinal fluid. Afterwards the two men, together with Lady Bruce and Gibbons who had both been admitted into the secret, proceeded to examine the cerebro-spinal fluid of thirty-four sleeping sickness patients. They found trypanosomes in twenty of these subjects, a figure which they inaccurately assessed as seventy per cent.

Castellani then wrote a somewhat reticent personal report on these findings which he despatched to the Royal Society on 5th April 1903, confident nevertheless that this would ensure his priority of discovery if later verified. On the same day, however, Bruce also sent off a letter informing the Society that he had 'helped' Castellani in his work, and indicated that the Italian would require recognition for his significant part in the epoch-making discovery – if he, Bruce, succeeded in substantiating it.

Castellani left for England next day, 6th April, and on 14th May his report (but not Bruce's letter) was read out before the Royal Society. Castellani's claim to priority was thus apparently enshrined.

He may have discovered the cause of sleeping sickness, but he had not indicated the method of its transmission, and it was to this subject that Bruce next turned his attention. Nabarro was now included in the research. Their work which followed was another model of scientific deduction. Bruce pondered over his experiments on nagana which had demonstrated that trypanosomes were transmitted by tsetse. He then persuaded local missionaries to report on the presence of fly in their parishes, and afterwards made a spot-map which clearly showed that their distribution matched that of sleeping sickness.

Bruce next allowed tsetse to feed on 'clean monkeys', and then duly noted the appearance of trypanosomes in their blood. Thus by 30th September the commission was able to report back to England that sleeping sickness was indeed 'conveyed from the sick to the healthy by tsetse flies', which they identified as *Glossina*. At the same time Bruce believed that this transmission was purely mechanical, on a soiled proboscis, and only several years later did he demonstrate that the trypanosome underwent development in the fly before it could be passed on to its human hosts.

The problem was solved, but the controversy over priority of revelation had scarcely begun. One person at least, Albert Cook, had no doubt as to where the credit lay; Bruce, he wrote, 'undoubtedly discovered the real cause of sleeping sickness, and Castellani of the first commission had been led off on quite the wrong scent.' Bruce was a shade less disparaging and reported correctly that Castellani had still been uncommitted to the incrimination of a trypanosome in sleeping sickness when the second commission arrived in Entebbe. Bruce did, however, go on to stress that it was his persuasion which had led the Italian to abandon his streptococcal theory and to concentrate instead on the trypanosome which he had previously considered to be no more than a contaminant.

Lankester and Manson became engaged in the unseemly dispute which followed, each man championing the merits of their protégés. It became a *cause célèbre*, but the passage of time has allowed us now to be less partisan. It seems fair to give Castellani the credit for discovering the parasites in patients suffering from trypanosomiasis, while Bruce placed Africa deeply in his debt for his recognition of the importance of the Italian's fortuitous discovery. But over the dispute there still hangs a cloud of sympathy for Nabarro who was denied his share in the fame gained at Entebbe by his two colleagues.

Castellani went on to enjoy an exciting career. After spending some time as Professor of Tropical Medicine in Ceylon, in 1915 he joined the Italian army when his native country entered the war on the side of the Allies. After serving with distinction on the Piave front he became a member of a medical commission to Poland, and was knighted by the King of England. Thereafter, Castellani established a fashionable practice in Harley Street until he assumed command of the Italian army medical services

during the Italo-Abyssinian conflict of 1935. He sub-
sequently resumed his military career as head of the health
services of the Italian forces in North Africa during the
Second World War and was ennobled by the King of Italy.
The discoverer of the cause of sleeping sickness, Professor
Marchese Sir Aldo Castellani died on 3rd October 1971.

By the end of 1903 it seemed only a matter of time before
the eradication of sleeping sickness would be effected. But it
gradually emerged that Bruce and Castellani had revealed
only a few of the problems about the disease, and many
more remained to be solved. Why for instance had it suddenly spread so dramatically? What therapeutic measures
could be devised to cure the established infection and what
means might be developed to exterminate tsetse fly in
Africa? To none of these questions has a completely convincing answer been given, and because both trypanosomes
and fly proved to be remarkably resistant to attack, sub-
Saharan Africa is still plagued by trypanosomiasis.
  Many interesting facts about these two mutual commensals which prey on man have, however, emerged from
massive research over the last seventy years. The fly is
clearly of very ancient origin. It is now believed to have
evolved from an ancestral insect living during the Carbon-
iferous Age some 260–230 million years ago. The flies
adapted to sucking reptiles' blood during the succeeding
Permian Age, and it has been suggested that they were then
responsible for the extinction of the dinosaurs which had
dominated animal life for so long. Certainly by the Eocene
Age, which began fifty-eight million years ago, few reptiles
were still living on land, apart from those like lizards, tor-
toises and snakes. The fly thus turned to prey on wild pigs,
and subsequently on elephants, rhinoceros, buffalo and
smaller kinds of buck. Over many millenia these animals
were able to adapt well to the trypanosome which had also
become parasitic on the blood-sucking tsetse flies. Game
animals in eastern Africa still provide a reservoir of these

blood parasites which in certain conditions will infect human beings. In western Africa game is more scarce and man provides the main trypanosome reservoir.

The name tsetse is of Tswana origin, another African word welcomed into English. It supposedly resembles the buzz of the insect. Elsewhere in Africa the fly is called chufwa and nsinsi which is said to sound like a fly's mating call. The Hausa named the fly tsande, a reference to its habit of preening itself. The scientific name for the tsetse is *Glossina* derived from the Greek for tongue, an allusion to the fly's large proboscis. *Glossina palpalis* and several related species transmit trypanosomiasis in western Africa; *G. morsitans* is the most common vector of the disease in savannah country east of the Great Rift Valley, where game is abundant. Unlike the mosquito both male and female flies prey on man and animals.

In savannah country the most common animal hosts for trypanosomes, and for the tsetse that ingest them, are small buck such as duiker and bushbuck. Other favoured hosts are buffalo, bush pig, warthog, sitatunga, giraffe, kudu and eland. In these animals the trypanosomes live a commensal-like existence. Carnivores are sometimes parasitised. Elsa the lion, heroine of *Born Free*, was found to harbour trypanosomes in her blood and Boy was actually treated for the condition. Domestic animals such as cattle, horses and exotic dogs are often fatally infected with *Trypanosoma brucei*. Donkeys and goats are less susceptible having acquired considerable immunity; they may take years to die of the disease, and Livingstone understandably believed that these animals did not suffer from nagana. Less popular with fly as food are hartebeest, waterbuck, impala, zebra, klipspringer, oribi, wildebeest, gazelles, stembok, leopard and hyena. Tsetse flies also bite reptiles, which harbour trypanosomes without harm to themselves. They particularly favour crocodile blood.

The tsetse does not lay eggs like most other insects. Instead a single fertilised egg develops into a larva within the fly's abdomen. This is then deposited on shady ground, immediately pupates, and over a five-week period matures into an adult fly.

After a fly's blood meal, any trypanosomes in the ingested blood multiply by simple longitudinal division and undergo development into infective forms which make their way to the insect's proboscis and salivary glands. It has been estimated that between three hundred and four hundred and fifty trypanosomes are injected each time an infected fly bites the animal prey. The number of bites sustained by the host is a vital consideration because there is evidence that man is capable of destroying about four hundred trypanosomes at a time, but the bodily defences are over-whelmed by a larger number. It appears that once infected during its first or second blood meal, a tsetse remains capable of transmitting trypanosomes for the remainder of its life-span, about two hundred days.

Morphological and pathogenic differences in the trypan-osomes responsible for the human disease have been closely studied. Two such species have been identified, but today they are considered by some authorities as merely separate strains. They are called *T. gambiense* and *T. rhodesiense*, the second of which occurs in patients in the eastern savannah. Both are virtually identical in appearance with *T. brucei* from which they are believed to have evolved and adapted in different degrees to parasitisation on man.

T. gambiense has affected human beings for so long in western Africa that man has developed some degree of tolerance to the organisms and the disease they cause is milder than that seen on the savannah; several years may pass before the trypanosomes let their weary prisoner die. Some patients make a partial recovery, though often with residual lethargy, deafness or mental retardation. After the tsetse has injected trypanosomes into the human body, they enter the blood stream causing headache, fever and pain in the limbs. They then migrate to the lymph glands, notably those in the neck; the patient now complains of weakness, his face swells and he is careless at work. The organisms subsequently invade that part of the brain which controls sleep, and eventually the patient is unable to look after himself, his skin becomes dry and covered with sores. Death follows lung inflammation, dysentery or starvation. *T. rhodesiense* is believed to be of comparatively recent origin and the disease it induces is more virulent.

Tsetse fly are mentioned several times in the Old Testament, notably in Isaiah VII, 18–25. Fly was correctly associated by Africans in the western part of the continent with sleeping sickness and nagana six hundred years ago, and the progress of the disease in a ruler of Mali was carefully recorded by an Arab traveller during the fourteenth century.

Many Africans were inclined to believe that human trypanosomiasis was caused by witchcraft, and a common curse was 'Owa na N'tola' – may you die of sleeping sickness. Those who were Moslems on the other hand suspected the disease to be punishment for apostasy. The disease became well known to European slavers on the Guinea Coast, who called it by various names including 'narcotic dropsy'. They recognised that the tell-tale swelling of the glands of the neck lowered the price of affected captives. During 1734 John Atkins, a naval surgeon, published an excellent account of the illness which he named 'the sleeping distemper'. He found that whipping and forced dancing failed to cure the sufferers' lethargy, and accordingly recommended bleeding, purging, snuff inhalation and sudden plunges into the cold sea. The listlessness and melancholy which accompanied the condition was ascribed by some slavers to homesickness rather than to an illness. The lethargy seen in so many captives on the West Coast gave the slavers the impression that all Africans were stupid and inept, and this in turn may have encouraged a feeling of superiority in the European.

South African voortrekkers during the 1830s encountered tsetse as they approached the Limpopo, and Africans living there informed them that fly caused the deaths of cattle and horses. They also indicated 'belts' of fly-free country, and told the Boers that cattle were not attacked by fly at night. As early as 1837 an English sportsman noted 'flies destructive to cattle' on his maps of the Limpopo region. David Livingstone, as we have seen, walked through thirty thousand miles of Africa without contracting trypanosomiasis or seeing it among the inhabitants, although he was well aware of the presence of nagana. It is clear that the human disease was then almost completely confined to the western part of the continent. During 1877 Timothy Lewis described trypanosomes in rats' blood and three years later Griffith Evans found similar parasites in camels suffering from a disease named Surra which investigations subsequently indicated was venereally transmitted. Bruce's recognition of the part played by the fly and blood fluke in nagana and sleeping sickness followed at the turn of the century.

We now know that small foci of the human disease smouldered in West Africa and the Congo basin for many centuries, and that the local Africans developed sufficient immunity to make their manifestations relatively mild. It was the European intrusion into Africa that led to one Congo focus rapidly expanding into new territory, its extension greatly assisted by the forty-eight steamers which were plying the great river by the turn of the century. Sir Roger Casement, who had recently joined the British Consular Service, was horrified by the impact of the disease on virgin communities: 'The population in the villages of Lukolela in 1891,' he wrote bitterly to the Belgian Governor-General, 'must have been not less than 6,000 people, but when I counted the whole population of Lukolela at the end of 1896 I found it to be only 719'. Joseph Conrad, who commanded a river steamer on the Congo during the early nineties, was equally appalled by the effect

of sleeping sickness on African labourers whom he encountered in a forest glade. In *Heart of Darkness* he wrote movingly
of the 'black shapes who crouched, lay, sat, between the
trees, leaning against the trunks, clinging to the earth, half
coming out, half effaced within the dim light, in all attitudes
of pain, abandonment and despair. . . . They were dying
slowly, nothing but black shadows of disease and starvation,
lying confusedly in the greenish gloom.' Presently the
disease reached Uganda and its impact startled even Dr
Albert Cook.

The outbreak of rinderpest during 1889–95 assisted the
expansion of human trypanosomiasis. It drastically reduced
the game in large parts of Africa, resulting in the tsetse flies
turning to man for food.

Medical treatment for sleeping sickness was ineffective
until the introduction of the synthetic drug atoxyl during
1904, but as Dr Schweitzer was to point out, it was 'frightfully
dangerous', its use often being followed by blindness. Since
then a succession of potent drugs such as tryparsamide,
suramin, pentamidine, furacin and malarsen have been
produced. Schweitzer was a pioneer in using tryparsamide
and after 1918 obtained good results. One of his early
patients was a forester named M'Tsama whose symptoms
included kleptomania, and Schweitzer was delighted to find
that a course of the new drug made an honest man of him. A
cure can be expected now in ninety per cent of early cases
treated in West Africa, and in about thirty per cent when the
disease is advanced. The figures are less favourable in
savannah cases, since the African patients there enjoy a
lesser degree of immunity to the infection. Chemoprophyl-
axis can be induced now against sleeping sickness by
injections of pentamidine given at six-monthly intervals.
Since 1949 antrycide has been used effectively to prevent
nagana in cattle.

Intense efforts have been made to eradicate tsetse fly
from Middle Africa and the struggle is one of the epics of
medical history. Following a conference held in London

during 1925 the British concentrated on the destruction of the fly's habitat through large scale bush clearing and destruction of shade vegetation, by organising somewhat ineffective gangs of fly-catchers, and by the trapping of tsetse in a number of ingenious contraptions. In addition, evacuation of the population from infected areas was sometimes enforced with excellent results, but this was highly unpopular with the people. Insecticides were subsequently used in enormous quantities for sleeping sickness control. Again, inital successes have been followed by disappointment in the long term. It was only gradually appreciated that the fly enjoys the same remarkable facility for breeding strains resistant to insecticides as does the mosquito. DDT also suffered the disadvantage of killing ants which feed on tsetse fly larvae.

Another approach to the control of sleeping sickness has been the widespread destruction of the game animals which act as reservoir hosts for trypanosomiasis. David Bruce was a particularly uncompromising advocate of killing off game in sleeping sickness areas, claiming that otherwise it would be as reasonable to 'allow mad dogs to live and be protected by law in our English towns and villages'. But game culling possesses grave disadvantages. The very absence of game tends to direct the fly to man, and in any case culling is repugnant to a conservation-minded public, and if carried to its logical conclusion would destroy one of Africa's greatest heritages.*

The French and Belgian colonial administrations attacked the problem in a different manner by treating all those suffering from the disease with full courses of tryparsamide, and giving smaller doses to all human contacts. The campaigns required close co-operation with the tribesmen, and when this was obtained it proved reasonably successful. But by the 1960s the system was in danger of breaking down

* A compromise may be reached by culling only the game whose blood is attractive to the tsetse, thus sparing hartebeest, water buck, impala and other animals.

as European public health staff were gradually withdrawn.

A more practical method of control has been evolved in Zimbabwe and elsewhere in Africa. A substance whose odour resembles that of the female tsetse fly's sex glands is used to entice males into suitable traps. There they are exposed to material which sterilises them. They are then released in quantities likely to exceed the number of un-treated male flies. As female tsetses mate only once in their lifetime and produce only a single larva at a time, this may effectively reduce the fly population. The method has the advantage of cheapness and the traps are easy to set up.

Efforts directed at the prevention of trypanosomiasis may thus be summarised as attempts at breaking man's contact with fly, direct destruction of fly, mass treatment of the human population at risk, and elimination of game. When put into practice all methods have resulted at first in a rapid reduction of the disease in both men and domestic animals, but this gain is rarely maintained. In a few years trypan-osomiasis usually returns as the fly and the blood parasite adapt to the new challenges.

The painstaking method of catching fly by hand is now rarely seen. Gone are the days when tattered regiments of 'fly boys' wearing white uniforms (after Schweitzer noted that fly tended not to pester people wearing white clothing) stalked through the bush with their nets and traps, to be paid each evening for the number of insects they had caught. Their successors are less numerous, but endowed with smarter uniforms and new dignity, being known as 'field assistants' and 'tsetse fly officers', but nevertheless still failing to win the fifty-year-old struggle against the bane of middle Africa.

The results of years of attempted eradication have been disappointing. Until the middle of this century the colonial powers seemed on the verge of suppressing human trypan-osomiasis and in doing so conferring on Africa one of the greatest blessings conceivable. In Nigeria, for instance, at the beginning of the century 11 per cent of the population was affected by the disease. By 1960 the figure had fallen to 0.15 per cent. In Zaire too it had been almost eliminated by 1960. But in both countries today the incidence is rising towards their old levels. For political disengagement by the colonial powers involved the replacement of a few but experienced administrations by numerous smaller states lacking funds, expertise in the field of preventive medicine, and inclination to co-operate on a pan-African scale. The civil disturbances which followed Independence have undoubtedly played a part too, in breaking down control methods, and in some African countries the intensity of research has diminished. But this is not the whole story. The adaptive capability of both the trypanosome and tsetse have been the chief cause for failure to control sleeping sickness in Black Africa.

Yet there are grounds for optimism. Cattle raising may usefully be replaced by ranching of game animals which are not affected by nagana, while special dwarf breeds of cattle which are immune to trypanosomiasis could be substituted for the larger animals which suffer from the disease. In the long term the outlook for human trypanosomiasis is heartening. More effective drugs will certainly be produced and the trypanosome is undoubtedly moving towards partnership with man. It must do so if it is to survive and we may look forward to the time when the trypanosomes cause no more trouble to human beings than they do to the game animals which shelter massive numbers of closely allied parasites without harm to themselves.

For the immediate future it is likely that greater emphasis will be replaced on the campaign against nagana than against human trypanosomiasis. The prizes are glittering. In Kenya alone, if fly could be brought under control, seven million square kilometres of grazing ground could be reclaimed, a very important gain to a continent whose people live always under the threat of starvation.

9

Yellow Fever

ON 15TH FEBRUARY, 1898, while Ronald Ross was on his way from the Kherwara 'convict station' to his triumphant work on bird malaria in Calcutta, he broke his journey at Agra to visit the Taj Mahal. Early that same morning an event occurred half a world away which was to lead to medical advances affecting Africa that would be almost as important as Ross's contribution. On that day the US battle-ship *Maine* blew up in Havana harbour, allegedly the victim of a mine laid by chauvinistic Spanish colonials in Cuba, with the loss of over two hundred American lives. Reaction in the United States was emotional and vigorous. Soon rampaging mobs were screaming 'to hell with Spain, remember *Maine*' through the streets of Washington, and the President was setting his signature to a document addressed to the King of Spain which was virtually a decla-ration of war.

The reasons for the conflict were in fact far more com-plex than the sinking of an American battleship. Ever since the end of the Civil War, the Americans had cherished ambitions to extend their country's influence throughout the Caribbean, and in a manner which hardly differed from those of the European imperialists whom they would later castigate with such fervour. Admittedly the war against Spain could be justified by the principles of the Monroe Doctrine, but other motives for the Americans' hostility existed. One of them was their determination to eradicate a mysterious disease of African origin which had gained a permanent hold in Cuba. From a focus in Havana, yellow fever had spread in a series of devastating epidemics to North America. New Orleans had suffered a savage outbreak during 1853; no less than fifteen epidemics struck Philadelphia alone during the eighteenth and nineteenth centuries, while New York was affected almost as frequently. During the single year, 1878, twenty-five thousand people died in the southern states from the disease. It was little wonder then that the Americans wished to control the slums of Havana in which epidemics were believed to originate.

The infection has as many as a hundred and fifteen different names. To mariners it was known as 'yellow jack', supposedly because of the quarantine flag flown from infected ships. Medical men preferred to call it 'yellow fever' since jaundice was one of its characteristic features. Various names referred to places of the scourge's origin like 'Bay of Benin fever'; others such as 'black vomit', indicated a prominent symptom while some like 'bilios remittent' were suggested by the course of the malady. The prevalence of yellow fever among wealthy tourists visiting Florida even caused it to be known as 'society fever', while the inhabitants of Latin America knew it gratefully as 'patriotic fever', since it had frequently succeeded in killing off foreign invaders.

Yellow fever does not fall among the first groups of tropical diseases which were categorised in chapter two, since Africans in endemic areas are highly resistant to the infection, but it is convenient to consider it here because, like malaria, filariasis and sleeping sickness, yellow fever is also transmitted by flying, biting insects.

When the United States went to war with Spain in 1898, the cause of yellow fever was a mystery, but Americans were convinced that if their country was to survive as a nation, the cesspit of infection in Havana must be eradicated. Certainly this was a factor that precipitated the Spanish-American conflict, one of the few wars that, to some extent at least, was initiated by a tropical illness.

The symptoms of yellow fever were reported by Portuguese mariners in West Africa during the fifteenth century, and accounts of fatal epidemics in Gambia go back as early as 1455. Inevitably the disease was confused with malaria although its symptoms are subtly different. Thus yellow fever runs a comparatively mild course in children who afterwards acquire a life-long immunity. Because most of the West Africans encountered by the early European mariners had accordingly gained immunity to yellow fever during childhood, the disease appeared primarily to affect expatriates. Only occasionally did it break through to affect Africans who lived outside an endemic area and thus lacked immunity.

The symptons of yellow fever are sudden and alarming. The patient complains of a wracking headache and is then prostrated by agonising pains. This is followed by the vomiting of large quantities of blood made greasy and black by the action of gastric juice. Half the victims of the infection simply vomit themselves to death within a few days. Those who recover retain immunity to the disease for life.

Until the cause of yellow fever was discovered, its treatment remained empirical. Bleeding was mandatory, while mercury, usually in the form of calomel, was regarded as 'the Samson of the *materia medica*' against the disease. Once an epidemic of yellow fever broke out, it was known to defy flight, fumigation and even cremation of corpses. It was particularly common among ships' companies but was recognised not to be contagious. This was once dramatically demonstrated to his shipmates on a yellow jack ship by a heroic doctor named McKinnial who publicly drank a wine-glassful of black vomit recently disgorged by a sick sailor. McKinnial then proceeded to allay the fears of his ship-mates by surviving his *geste*.

White expatriates living on the Guinea Coast dreaded epidemics of yellow fever, particularly as the disease spared most Africans there. The experiences of Europeans in Gambia were typical of those resident in other colonies like Senegal, Sierra Leone and Ghana. As already noted, a disease which can be identified as yellow fever was mentioned in Gambia during 1455. After the British occupation of 1816 seventy-four men from the Bathurst garrison of one hundred and five soldiers died from the disease. Then in 1837 half the European population of Bathurst died from another outbreak which had been brought there from Sierra Leone in HMS *Curlew*. Subsequent epidemics occurred in 1842, 1859, 1866 and 1878 (when thirteen out of fifty white residents died). The next epidemic broke out during 1900, and it is noteworthy because during it the possibility of mosquito transmission was first mooted in the settlement. During a later epidemic, that of 1934, panic seized Bathurst; all the white women were evacuated to England and the men to Cape St Mary, while preventive measures were taken, including the stripping of gutters from all houses and the felling of five thousand trees. The tragic story of yellow fever in Bathurst was repeated along the coast.

The geographical origin of yellow fever was for many years the subject of wide debate. The fifteenth-century report from Gambia of a lethal fever which differed in its manifestations from malaria had been forgotten when repeated outbreaks of yellow fever occurred in the New World during the seventeenth century. These all suggested that the disease was of American origin. In fact, until 1778 most cases of yellow fever in West Africa were diagnosed as malaria. Only after this date was yellow fever finally accepted as different, and naturally it was then assumed to be an import from America.

Modern research, however, has now confirmed that yellow fever originated in Africa. Its distribution in western Africa has been mapped out by the mouse protection test. The method of this test is to inject yellow fever virus into mice, together with a small amount of human blood. If that blood is taken from someone who has already suffered from yellow fever, his antibodies against the disease will protect the mouse and it will survive the experiment. On the other hand if the human subject has never had the disease, the mouse will die.

Campaigns to define the endemic areas of yellow fever by means of this test demonstrated that many people in much of West Africa possess immunity to the disease. The region of yellow fever immunity stretches from the southern border of the Sahel to Angola and as far east as the Great Rift Valley. The population of this enormous expanse of country can only have gained this protection from child-hood infections. These findings came as a surprise, but they provided convincing evidence that yellow fever was a disease of African origin, since this high degree of immunity could have been gained only over the course of many centuries.

The general consensus today is that the virus of yellow fever was carried from Africa across the Atlantic following Columbus's discovery of America; and other facts, apart from the earlier identification of the disease in Gambia, support this proposition: several species of *Aedes* mosquitoes which transmit yellow fever, exist in Africa, but only one in America, and a larger species variation would almost certainly have occurred had this not been a recent immigrant; and finally many of the Caribbean islands remained free from the disease for more than a hundred years after their discovery during the fifteenth century.

The infected agents of yellow fever which were ferried to the Americas were mosquitoes of the *Aedes* genus. These mosquitoes are highly domestic, haunting human living quarters especially aboard ships, where open water containers present them with ideal breeding places. Surviving the Atlantic crossing they infected the Amerindians who lacked all natural protection to yellow fever and died at an alarming rate. The range of infection increased as more mosquitoes carrying the disease arrived in America during the long years of the Atlantic slave trade. The *Aedes* bred rapidly in their new environment and local allied strains of mosquitoes took up the infection. The stage was thus set for the devastating epidemics which periodically swept Central America and endangered the future of the United States.

Further research in Africa has shown that yellow fever is a
disease of monkeys as well as of men, and since time
immemorial these have provided a massive reservoir
of infection. This reservoir ensured that almost all the
Africans living in an endemic area became infected as
children and thus acquired permanent immunity after a
mild illness. It is only recently that effective eradication of
Aedes from many regions has allowed large numbers of
Africans to escape the disease during childhood, so they are
now at risk if new epidemics break out following relaxation
of mosquito control.

Ships carrying yellow jack were greatly feared. Crewmen
incubating the disease before sailing would infect mosquito
fellow-travellers. These in turn bit healthy sailors who
would sicken, and in due course most of the crew became
affected. Ships carrying the infection flew a warning yellow
flag and many ports would deny them entry. One such ship
was the legendary *Flying Dutchman* which haunts the seas
round the Cape of Good Hope, its crew forever seeking
sanctuary in some friendly harbour. Sightings of the *Dutchman* are still reported and reputed to bring bad luck. The
ship's eternal spectral voyage so caught at public imagination that Marryat wrote a novel and Wagner an opera on
the subject, while Coleridge's *Ancient Mariner* is based in part
on the fable.

Yellow fever exerted a profound effect on world history. It repeatedly defeated European incursions into the
Americas. Thus it frustrated a British attempt to colonise
Puerto Rico in 1598 after its capture from the Spanish by
Lord Cumberland's army. Within five months the disease
had destroyed the army of occupation and the remnants
abandoned the new colony. A century and a half later,
during the War of Jenkins' Ear, the same disease killed off
two thirds of the British forces besieging Cartagena, and the
surviving troops were hastily evacuated.

Yellow fever gained its most significant military victory
against the army which Napoleon sent to seize Saint Dom-

ingo during 1801. It was commanded by his brother-in-law, General Leclerc, and numbered thirty-three thousand men. The intention was to use Haiti as a base from which the French would strengthen their existing hold on the Mississippi valley. But yellow fever killed twenty-nine thousand of the soldiers and only a sickly remnant of the expeditionary force returned to Europe. Thereafter, Napoleon abandoned his ambitions in the New World, selling the state of Louisiana and the surrounding country to the infant American republic.

Yellow fever has never affected Asia although suitable mosquito vectors abound there. It was feared that it only needed a single infected mosquito to reach Asia from Africa to set off a devastating epidemic, but gradually it became appreciated that the insects could not survive the cold sea passages round South Africa or South America. With the construction of the Panama Canal, however, all the old fears of the disease reaching Asia were renewed. Fortunately no spread of infection occurred, not even after the introduction of fast air communications. To account for this deliverance it has been suggested (though by no means generally accepted) that there is a limit to the number of separate viruses which can establish themselves in a given area, and that the Asiatic mosquitoes, already carrying their full complement, can accept no more.

A long dispute concerned the cause of yellow fever. As in the case of malaria it was commonly attributed to 'diffusable miasma' or to contaminated water. So strongly did two medical practitioners feel about their differing opinions that they fought a duel, in which both were killed. Other authorities claimed that the fever followed inhalation of vapour liberated from newly turned soil, while Dr Benjamin Rush, who nursed Philadelphia through the epidemic of 1793, was certain that the responsible poison emanated from rotting coffee beans left lying on the wharves.

The suggestion that mosquitoes carried the disease was first put forward in 1848 by another American, Dr Josia

Nott, who as we have seen, also tentatively incriminated mosquitoes as the vectors of malaria. But his theory had been forgotten thirty years later when Dr Carlos J. Finlay, who was thereafter referred to by his colleagues as 'that crazy Cuban doctor', propounded the same hypothesis. The son of a French mother and a Scots physician who had settled in Cuba, Finlay practised medicine in Havana. There, in over a hundred experiments, he fed *Aedes* mosquitoes on volunteers, and awaited the results. Finlay had not appreciated that the insects did not become infective for some days after ingesting the virus, and in consequence only a few of his volunteers in fact went down with yellow fever. But on the strength of this qualified result Finlay felt able, on 14th August 1881, to read a paper on his theory of mosquito transmission to an audience of sleepy and unimpressed Academicians in Havana. He went on to suggest that ships' cisterns and water containers provided admirable breeding places for the mosquitoes which carried the disease, and emphasised that this explained the occurrence of 'fever ships'. Though no one took 'that crazy doctor' Finlay's work very seriously, he persisted in writing articles to support his conclusions. In addition he published methods of mosquito control and indicated a geographical relationship between the incidence of yellow fever and the distribution of *Aedes* mosquitoes, these observations being all the more remarkable because news of Manson's work on the transmission of filariasis by mosquitoes had still to reach Cuba. Finlay also identified a bacillus which he said caused the disease. It was his only mistake.

When American soldiers occupied Cuba towards the end of the Spanish War, many of them succumbed to yellow fever. At this time Finlay was still practising in Havana, and, having learned of Ross's results, he was more than ever certain that *Aedes* transmitted yellow fever. He welcomed the American decision to deal with the crisis by appointing a board of army doctors comprising Major Walter Reed, James Carroll and Jesse Lazear to investigate the fever.

These officers presently met Finlay and found him to be 'a lovable man' who was anxious to be helpful. To begin with, Reed scoffed at Finlay's theories and it was only after two months' delay that he decided to test them. Finlay obligingly supplied the board with *Aedes* eggs, and he was enrolled on its staff together with a Cuban colleague, Aristedes Agramonte.

In the absence of known animal hosts for the disease, Reed decided to use human volunteers in his investigations. The majority were Spanish and Irish immigrants on the island who were in fact paid for 'volunteering', while the numbers were made up by American soldiers acting under orders. James Carroll offered himself as one of the human guinea pigs, and on 27th August 1900, after several attempts with *Aedes* mosquitoes, he and another soldier were successfully infected with yellow fever. Both men recovered. A little later Lazear allowed a mosquito that settled on his arm to bite him. He presently sickened with yellow fever and died. It was a sad loss, but the tragedy removed most of the doubts about the transmission of the disease.

The board reacted energetically to the new situation. Reed settled seven Americans in a mosquito-screened hut, to sleep there using linen and pillows taken from the beds of recent yellow fever victims. None of them went down with the disease. Here was positive proof that the disease was not contagious, and disinfection of patients unnecessary.

Next, a screened hut was set up with two compartments. Fifteen infected *Aedes* mosquitoes were introduced into one section together with a single volunteer. After four days the volunteer developed yellow fever. Men living in the adjoining compartment remained healthy. Mosquito transmission of the disease was thereafter accepted as proven.

Further experiments demonstrated that mosquitoes do not become infective until twelve days after feeding on a yellow fever patient, while humans became briefly infective two or three days after being bitten. Their blood remained infective even after being passed through a filter fine enough to prevent the passage of bacteria, an indication that the infecting germ was a virus, although this conclusion was not immediately accepted.

The board's findings were made known on 23rd October 1900, and the part played by *Aedes* transmission was subsequently confirmed in both Africa and Central America.

Even before he had positively identified the vector of yellow fever, Reed developed a plan to rid Havana of its burden of disease. He chose another American army doctor, William Crawford Gorgas, to put his ideas into effect. By one of those coincidences which so often enliven history, Gorgas was brought into the world by the same Josia Nott who had been the first to suggest that yellow fever was transmitted by a mosquito. Gorgas's family was living in Charleston when the American Civil War broke out during 1861, and he would later speak about his memories of the bombardments of Fort Sumpter which sparked off hostilities. His father soon resigned his federal commission and joined the southern forces. His subsequent brilliant military career made young Gorgas long to follow him into the army, but he failed to enter West Point and found he could only hope to become a soldier by training as a doctor. Gorgas duly qualified during 1880 and promptly entered the Army Medical Corps. While serving in Texas he survived a sharp attack of yellow fever, and since it was known that this provided immunity to the disease, volunteered for service in Cuba when the Spanish War broke out. Reed placed him in charge of the sanitary control of the newly captured city of Havana.

Believing that yellow fever was a 'filth disease', Gorgas applied himself first to cleaning up the city. He improved its garbage disposal and refashioned a medieval drainage system. But although these measures were followed by a dramatic fall in the incidence of malaria, typhoid and dysentery, they made no impression on yellow fever, which in fact raged more violently than ever during 1900.

Soon afterwards, Reed's demonstration of the mosquito transmission of the disease made Gorgas change his tactics. He screened and fumigated the soldiers' quarters in Havana and those of all civilians who went down with it. Then he turned to the control of *Aedes* breeding places, eliminating all static water, and applying stringent penalties to those who failed to do so on private premises. In addition he used vast quantities of oil to destroy mosquito larvae and for good measure introduced fish to eat any living in open water. His results were highly successful and they set Reed writing to him, 'You have succeeded in throttling the epidemic . . . it is to your everlasting credit.' By the end of the year yellow fever had been banished from Havana. Soon afterwards the whole of Cuba was free, and after 1909 no more cases were reported from the United States. Preventive medicine had won one of its most impressive triumphs.

Confident that it was now possible to control mosquitoes in any specified area, the American government presently felt justified in considering the building of a ship canal across the isthmus of Panama. This damp, tropical jungle was recognised as one of the unhealthiest places on earth. Malaria and yellow fever were endemic and their combined presence twenty years earlier had defeated the bid by Ferdinand de Lesseps, fresh from his triumphant completion of the Suez canal, to link the Atlantic and Pacific Oceans. During the nine years following 1881, de Lesseps had lost three quarters of his European employees in Panama from mosquito-borne disease, while the locally recruited labourers perished in such numbers that it was said that there remained 'hardly enough trees in the isthmus for crosses to mark their graves'.

Having decided to make a canal, the US government discovered that the most suitable site lay within Colombian territory. This difficulty was, however, quickly overcome by methods repeated in various places later. A revolution was fomented among the inhabitants of the isthmus, the Colombian troops which were called in were restrained by

American soldiers from crushing the rising, and a new Panamanian state was proclaimed. A land concession was then extracted from the infant independent nation which would permit the digging of a canal from Panama City to Colon, and which would remain under effective American control.

With political difficulties thus satisfactorily eliminated, Gorgas during 1904 was placed in medical charge of the workers who were to construct the new canal. He proceeded to launch a sanitary compaign which became a model for all future attempts to eradicate disease from the tropics. He was fortunate in having at his disposal a large annual budget. He used it to screen all dwelling places in the canal zone and then methodically fumigated them with pyrethrum, while a small army of labourers were recruited to eliminate mosquito breeding places. Clean water containers were set up wholesale to entice mosquitoes to lay their eggs where they could be easily destroyed, and forested lands surrounding the canal were systematically destroyed by fire. During the first two years of construction, however, fifty-seven Americans working in the zone died from yellow fever or malaria and in one particularly bad three-month period, five hundred Americans quit their jobs on the canal. After Gorgas's measures became effective, not a single death from these diseases occurred.

As with Ross, Gorgas's work was greatly hampered by superiors' criticism of his methods, and on several occasions he was threatened with dismissal. This was the fate of many successful sanitary pioneers, but the more fortunate Gorgas was saved by Presidential intervention.

The canal was triumphantly completed in 1914 after an estimated three million dollars had been expended in clearing a tiny strip of land of mosquitoes. But for Gorgas's work it was accepted that the Americans would have lost four thousand men from disease with thirteen thousand of their work force constantly in hospital. Gorgas had shown that with sufficient financial resources, tropical diseases

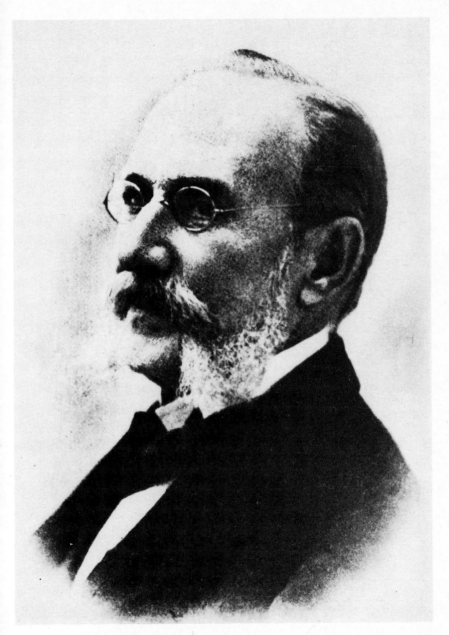
5 Carlos Juan Finlay (1833–1915) – Finlay practised medicine in Havana and was one of the first men to suspect the transmission of yellow fever by mosquitoes

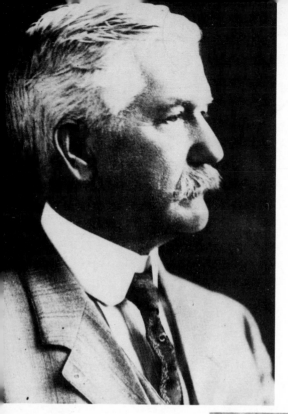

6 William Crawford Gorgas (1854–1920) – Gorgas served in Cuba during the Spanish American War of 1898 and subsequently eliminated yellow fever in Havana. In 1904 he became Chief Sanitary Officer of the Panama Canal project and eradicated malaria and yellow fever from the area thus making work on the canal possible

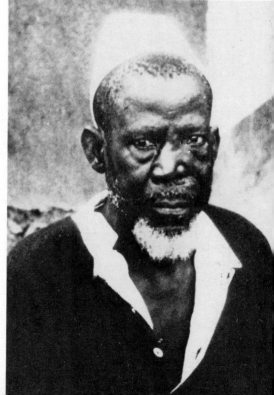

7 Asibi, an African labourer in Ghana, who was infected with yellow fever. The virus from his blood was attenuated and the strain used to produce a yellow fever vaccine which is still in use today

could be eliminated from a limited area, but it left medical men elsewhere wondering uneasily how much money it would require to clear away the whole burden of illness from sub-Saharan Africa.

When Gorgas visited Great Britain in 1913 he was well received; Osler described his reception at the Royal Society of Medicine as 'the greatest ever accorded to a medical man in England', while the *Daily Mail* eulogised Gorgas with 'perhaps of all living Americans, he has conferred the greatest benefits on the human race'. Like Castellani, Gorgas was knighted by King George V. He died in London in 1920 while on his way to investigate the incidence of yellow fever in the Congo. When a memorial service was held for him at St Paul's, the only floral tribute allowed on his bier came from Sir Patrick Manson.

Though the vector of yellow fever had been positively identified before the Panama Canal was built, the nature of the organism responsible for the disease had still to be discovered. From time to time a new bacillus would be incriminated, the most favoured candidate being hopefully named *Bacillus icteroides* but none passed their tests. Then in 1924 a well-known Japanese scientist, Hideyo Noguchi, claimed that he had solved the problem after finding a spirochaete in the blood of several patients whom he thought were suffering from yellow fever. But parallel experiments failed to confirm Noguchi's findings. Noguchi presently took himself off to West Africa to do more work on the disease. There it was said he inoculated himself with blood from a yellow fever case to prove his theory, or perhaps in a spirit of hari-kari. Whatever his reason, Noguchi, no less than Lazear, died a martyr to the conquest of yellow fever. The colleague who conducted an autopsy on him, in turn became infected and died. The toll of the mysterious disease among its scientific enemies was increasing.

It was not until 1927 that Adrian Stokes was able to demonstrate that the causal organism of the disease was a filter-passing virus which was harmless to its insect vectors.

His research had been financed by the Rockefeller Foundation, which besides many other philanthropic activities had undertaken a programme to study yellow fever. Stokes and his colleagues also succeeded in infecting rhesus monkeys with the virus, so that human volunteers could now be dispensed with for their experiments. Stokes himself died from yellow fever after becoming infected while conducting an autopsy; he had omitted the usual precaution of putting on rubber gloves to prevent accidental infection through unnoticed abrasions in the skin of the hands.

Now that the transmitter and causal agent of yellow fever had been recognised it was hoped that mosquito destruction would control the disease. The results proved disappointing, for the habits of the *Aedes* mosquitoes differ from those of the anopheline: the *Aedes* are domestic insects which breed in artificial containers rather than in naturally occurring water. Neither clearing areas of pools and puddles nor the provision of proper drainage, therefore, affect them. They prefer to lay their eggs in such unlikely places as flower pots and empty cans which are unlikely to be reached by gangs spraying insecticides.

Control is also rendered difficult because yellow fever is essentially a disease of monkeys which provide an inexhaustible reservoir of infection. To make matters worse, one strain of the virus parasitises mosquitoes which live, like many monkeys, in the high canopy of trees in heavily forested areas of Africa and they are not of the *Aedes* group. Occasionally infected 'jungle' mosquitoes bite forest dwellers and the infection may then be continued by *Aedes*, the usual carrier. Jungle outbreaks of yellow fever are rare but its control is almost impossible in areas which are difficult to penetrate.

Gradually it became apparent that only the production of a yellow fever vaccine would be likely to control the disease. Fortunately, while working on another programme funded by the Rockefeller Foundation, Dr A.F. Mahaffy was able to develop just such a safe and stable protective vaccine.

He collected blood from an African labourer named Asibi who was suffering from yellow fever and succeeded in 'passing'* the responsible virus through a series of monkeys and subsequently mice. This resulted in this virus losing its toxic effects on man in a process named 'attenuation'. By 1932 an effective vaccine had come into use which was derived from the original Asibi strain of the virus. This was the only strain that has been thus attenuated. The work was carried out in the Rockefeller Institute, New York.

Vaccinations campaigns against yellow fever were then introduced in western and in central Africa among communities at risk. One injection was found to protect a person from the infection for at least five years.

Yellow fever had therefore seemingly joined those other human diseases which are totally preventable. Asibi derived no benefit from his unqiue contribution to the control of yellow fever until Mahaffy several years later paid him a visit in Ghana. Mahaffy found Asibi to be in poor health and circumstances. His assurances to Asibi that he had helped large numbers of people throughout the world failed to comfort him but Mahaffy's representations subsequently led to a government pension being granted to him.

Unfortunately, the lowering of the incidence of yellow fever which followed mass vaccination was not permanent. After independence some of the new African countries were simply unable to afford to continue the campaigns or to maintain vigilance teams who would report new outbreaks of the infection. In Senegal mass vaccination against yellow fever was abandoned during 1960, and a severe outbreak followed in 1965. Other devastating epidemics of yellow fever have since occurred in western Africa, though the resulting mortality was not adequately appreciated because of poor surveillance and official reluctance to

* 'passing' in this context means that a monkey is inoculated with the yellow fever virus and its infection is artifically continued through the inoculation of a succession of other monkeys until the virus loses its toxicity.

publish figures. An epidemic in unvaccinated Gambia during June 1978 resulted in only thirty cases being notified, though subsequent serum testing suggested that eight thousand four hundred people were infected, of whom one thousand six hundred died.

Nor has the introduction of Mahaffy's vaccine affected the incidence of jungle yellow fever in Africa. Although this variety of the disease is generally mild amongst forest dwellers who possess some immunity, the unvaccinated inhabitants of savannah land adjoining forest areas are believed to be at risk from the infection.

The danger of spreading the yellow fever virus out of Africa increased with the growing use of air travel, but effective action has been taken by the compulsory vaccination of travellers and the fumigation of aircraft passing through endemic areas. Failure to preserve the rigorous standards of yellow fever control would result in the spread of the disease in the Americas as well as in its native Africa with serious consequences.

10

Bilharzia –
the Egyptian Inheritance

THE ENDING OF the Second World War again deposited our family on the shores of Lake Nyasa, this time at Nkhotakota which lies about one hundred and fifty kilometres north of the old dispensary at Kachindomoto.

Because of its situation, Moslem population and surrounding paddy fields, Nkhotakota was the very capital of bilharzia in Nyasaland. This disease is caused by human parasitic blood flukes, and it rivals malaria and sleeping sickness in being the greatest threat to human health in tropical Africa, yet it is rarely a lethal disease; rather it is the continent's largest purveyor of human debility.

The fluke – a comparatively large flat worm – was described as early as 1851 by a German named Theodor Bilharz after he noticed one during an autopsy carried out in Cairo. It is a bisexual organism which permits a useful division of labour. The bulky male parasite concentrates on providing protection for the flimsier female worm, whose main function is reproductive.

The female measures some two centimetres in length; the male is about half as long. Manson's friend, the entomologist Spencer Cobbold, gave the parasite and the disease it carries the names of bilharzia and bilharziasis after its discoverer, but purists subsequently claimed that the worm had already been called schistosomia by another scientist. Both synonyms are in use, although by the rules of biological nomenclature priority is given to schistosoma and schistosomiasis. We, on the lake, were inclined to use 'bilharzia' for both the fluke and the illness, and usually spoke of the commoner urinary form as 'Bill Harry'* which seemed to roll off the tongue more easily than the sibiliant 'schistosomiasis'. The condition also goes under the name of endemic haematuria (bleeding during urination) and 'snail fever', which provides an indication of the parasite's intermediate host.

Different species of the fluke cause three main forms of the disease; two occur in Africa, the third in the Far East. Of the African varieties, *Schistosoma mansoni* inhabits man's intestinal blood vessels and causes dysenteric symptoms. Although causing a more severe illness, it is less prevalent than the *S. haematobium*, the urinary form, which is accordingly a far greater obstacle to the continent's development.

The male and female flukes which cause urinary bilharzia usually affect peasant populations especially those in close contact with water. These small worms, like all parasites, are very logical organisms. Their own survival depends on keeping their human hosts alive, yet at the same time they must reduce them to such lethargy and apathy as to be incapable of finding ways to cast off their parasitic yokes. The flukes achieve this by causing a persistent loss of blood into the bladder, prolonged parasitic competition for nourishment, and through the destructive effect of those of their eggs which lodge in human tissues. These factors combine to cause chronic infirmity.

The numerical facts about bilharzia are horrifying. Its three species are estimated to affect over two hundred million persons. About fifty million black Africans suffer from the urinary disease and many of them also harbour the intestinal fluke. Worse, the prevalence of bilharzia is rapidly increasing in Africa. It is one of the continent's tragedies that the very measures taken to improve her people's quality of life are precisely those which have added to the burden of this infection. Every irrigation scheme which is planned and every dam built inevitably brings the African peasants into

* The name also reminded us nostalgically of 'Bell Harry', the great tower of Canterbury Cathedral.

new contact with the snails that carry bilharzia. Every bridge constructed and each new house is likely to be associated with the formation of artificial pools of water which provide homes for the snails that carry and maintain the disease.

The male and female flukes which cause bilharzia in the urinary form live together in the veins draining the human bladder. In them they mate periodically and in mating the leaf-like body of the male forms itself into an elongated groove which embraces its threadlike female partner. On becoming pregnant the female worm moves down the vein, against the blood flow towards the bladder. When the veins narrow it can go no further, the mother fluke discharges numerous showers of fertilised eggs.

The eggs are sharply pointed and this helps them to penetrate the bladder wall. The passage is further assisted by contractions of the bladder and the eggs' secretion of a digestive juice. Nevertheless the penetration of the bladder is traumatic and responsible for bleeding, distressing inflammatory changes and residual scarring. The first sign of the infection is accordingly the passage of bloody urine. Later on the disease may be complicated by the formation of stones and polyps in the bladder, and the latter sometimes become cancerous.

A large proportion of the eggs fail to work their way through the bladder wall and remain unhatched in the body. These errant eggs are washed back into the host's general bloodstream and are scattered throughout the patient's system where they presently die. The piling up of dead eggs blocks the normal flow of body fluid through the vital organs, and they act too as irritating foreign bodies which results in localised formation of fibrous tissue as the host attempts to wall them off. The fibrosis in turn leads to all manner of clinical complications. Thus ova which lodge in the brain often cause epilepsy, which in Black Africa usually presents itself as extensive burns because of its victims' liability during fits to fall into the open fires maintained in their huts. (In this context it is interesting to note that epilepsy is much feared by the Africans, and some of them believe it to be contagious.) As the number of eggs in the body increases astronomically, many are deposited in the liver which develops cirrhosis, and the patient becomes weak and emaciated. All this time bilharzial eggs are constantly being discharged when their host urinates, and many will be passed into fresh water. For human beings have a predilection for urinating in water, especially if water plants provide some degree of privacy (this being particularly true of Mohammedans who customarily cleanse themselves after urinating). Fresh water is vital for the bilharzial eggs, for only in it will their protective shells rupture and release free-swimming larvae called miracidia.

The miracidia at once seek out a particular fresh-water snail whose body, if they are to survive, they must enter by active penetration. Once safely within the snail the miracidia give rise to many arrow-shaped progeny named cercariae. These larval forms are scarcely visible to the naked eye, but can be readily seen with a hand lens. During a single month one miricidium is believed capable of producing one hundred thousand free-swimming cercariae.

Again in the bilharzial cycle one is astonished at the reproductory waste of nature, for only very few cercariae will survive to find a human host and complete their cycle. They are strong swimmers and their biological objective is to find and enter human flesh. Their search is facilitated by the attraction exerted by their prey's bodily heat and also by the sebum from man's sebacious glands. Their victims are people who come to fresh water pools to work, bathe, drink, wash clothes and for excretary purposes. They are reinfected almost daily as they paddle through infested water which they may also use as privies and so keep the parasite cycle turning incessantly. These people become riddled with parasite eggs, and a brisk haemorrhage from the bladder in boys where bilharzia is endemic is regarded, like menstruation, as a sign of puberty. The victims' bellies swell to accommodate a damaged, swollen liver; energy is replaced

by apathy; the community becomes weighed down by its
load of parasites and its industry languishes. Worse, a
vicious circle sets in: less food is grown by these tired people;
they come to suffer increasingly from malnutrition and lose
hope of finding ways to rid themselves of their parasitic
yoke.

The odds against cercariae making contact with a human
being during their two-day life-span were high enough in
most regions to justify the flukes' exuberant fertility, but at
Nkhotakota and in other villages on the shores of Lake
Nyasa they were offered whole regiments of human hosts.
Once these had been located, the cercariae usually penetrate
the skin of the foot or leg (though a small proportion enter
the body in drinking water). Having burrowed through the
skin the infant flukes shed their 'tails' and pass into the
human bloodstream. Some six weeks later their new host
experiences an explosive onset of high fever, general bodily
pains and weakness. These symptoms are due to the body's
allergic response to the flukes' foreign protein injected into
its system. As the temperature subsides the disease enters its
more serious, chronic stage. For having made an intracor-
poreal pilgrimage, whose complexity rivals that of the hookworm, the bilharzial flukes finally reach their intended
living place in the veins, draining their new host's bladder.
There the worms mature into male and female forms, and
the whole involved cycle begins again.

The bilharzia flukes boast a long ancestry. They infected
the ancient Egyptians, and typical eggs have been recovered
from mummies dating back to 1500 BC. Moreover papyri
several times mention various forms of treatment for a
disease characterised by bloody urine which was almost
certainly bilharzia. Wars and migrations carried the flukes
from the Nile valley to the central African lakes whence this
inheritance from Egypt became distributed through most
of the continent. The Mosaic warnings concerning the
drinking of impure water are believed to have been directed
at the prevention of bilharzia and guinea-worm infections.

Europe first learned about bilharzia after Bonaparte's expedition into Egypt during 1798. His soldiers soon began to suffer severely from a disease characterised by the painful passing of bloody urine. A century later bilharzia became such a problem to British troops serving against the Boers that for years Whitehall annually paid out £10,000 to soldiers incapacitated by the disease (some of whom were still passing eggs as late as 1920, an indication of the fluke's longevity).

The bilharzia fluke appears to have a talent for harassing the military. When the Americans stormed ashore on Leyte in October 1944 they encountered these same animal parasites, about which, incredibly, they had received no warning. Symptoms of the infection did not appear immediately, and it was only on New Year's Day 1945 that the first military cases were diagnosed among patients in an evacuation hospital. In the end one thousand seven hundred men were put out of action by the fluke, at a cost of three hundred thousand fighting-man-days and three million dollars. The lesson of the dangers from bilharzia had not been learned five years later then fifty thousand Chinese communist soldiers assembled during 1950 for the projected invasion of Formosa. Bilharzia became widespread among them and led to the abandonment of the campaign and the survival of Chiang Kai-Shek's island nation of Taiwan.

More than any other infection, bilharzia is an arithmetical disease, in that the severity of its symptoms and the cumulative damage it causes to the host's body are directly related to the number of flukes harboured by each patient. In heavy infections the adult parasites may number several hundreds. The maturing flukes live in something close to symbiosis with their human hosts; the varied symptoms of bilharzia are caused later by their eggs which either directly injure the bladder or lie scattered throughout the internal organs where they act as irritating, obstructive foreign substances.

Over the centuries the inhabitants of Black Africa, often in daily exposure to it, developed some degree of immunity to the harmful effects of bilharzia infection. Europeans, however, with no such immunity display far more severe symptoms while often carrying a lighter parasitic load.

The highest incidence of infection occurs in African children, although the parasites may still be too few to cause obvious clinical signs. At Nkhotakota I found eggs present in fifty-one per cent of urine samples taken from two thousand children, and the figure significantly increased when several specimens were examined. Infection was seen in very few infants under three years, presumably because they had not been exposed to snail habitats. The number of infected boys slightly exceeded that of girls.In some parts of Africa an infection rate of ninety-eight per cent has been reported. The incidence decreases with age; thus during 1960 one survey team reported that twenty per cent of Tanganyikan children were infected while barely ten per cent of adults were passing eggs. Such a finding suggests either that childhood infection later contributes to a high mortality or that after some twenty years exposure to the fluke, some infected persons develop the means to destroy their parasitic loads.

Bilharzia figures from African states between 1934 and 1957 were of great concern to the medical authorities. During this period some parts of Ghana reported a seventy per cent occurrence in children, Nigeria over eighty per cent, Zambia eighty-two per cent and Zaire sixty-three per cent. There is good evidence that the incidence of the disease is now rising in some parts of Africa, those at particular risk being rice growers, fish farmers and workers on irrigation projects.

It has already been noted that bilharzia is not an immediately dangerous disease like malaria and sleeping sickness; it is the long-term debilitating effect the infection exerts on its hosts which presents so great a menace to the future well-being of Africa. But because bilharzia rarely occurs as an acute and fatal infection, little research into the origin of the disease was mounted until long after the causes of the more deadly infections were discovered. This is all the more remarkable since an association between fresh water snails and bilharzia had long been suspected. As early as the 1880s that odd genius, Emin Pasha, when marooned for years in Central Africa, actually incriminated one particular snail as the vector of bilharzia. To honour the man who rescued him, Emin named this snail *Biomphalaria alexandrina stanlei.** Several other fresh water snails have since been identified as intermediate hosts of bilharzia. All favour slow-flowing, fresh-water streams, pools, shallows of lakes, dams, ditches and irrigation furrows.

British troops serving in Egypt during the First World War suffered so severely from the disease that they provided the impetus which led to scientific research into its origin. A serving doctor, R.T. Leiper, had already learned a good deal about oriental schistosomiases while working in Japan, and he was hastily despatched to deal with the medical crisis in the Nile delta. He knew that shaven mice could be infected with bilharzia and in a very short time, using these animals as experimental hosts, he had worked out the whole bilharzial cycle and advised on elementary methods of snail control. His results were published in the *Journal of the Royal Army Medical Corps* no doubt to the great gratification of Sir David Bruce who by then had become Commandant of the Millbank Hospital.

The development of an effective treatment for bilharzia infection proved a large problem, and it was not until 1918 that tartar emetic injections were shown to be reasonably effective in killing the adult flukes. But the therapy possessed two shortcomings; it entailed a prolonged course of intravenous injections, and they often provoked severe side effects. Its toxicity and the need for highly trained staff to administer the drug made it unsuitable for mass treatment

* Science has since prescribed a less evocative name for this snail, leaving us still guessing at the identity of Alexandrina.

campaigns in Africa, especially as few patients were likely to complete the prescribed course of painful injections.

No account of the discovery of the fluke's cycle and early treatment would be complete without some mention of the work of an heroic American doctor named Barlow. To prove the method of bilharzia transmission to man, Dr C. Barlow placed two hundred and twenty-four live cercariae on his belly and waited patiently for a succession of nettle-like stings to announce the entry of the bilharzia larvae into his skin. He presently went down with a severe bilharzial infection which demanded so many injections of tartar emetic that, in his old age, Barlow wrote, 'even today I shudder every time I see a hypodermic needle.'

It was not until 1948 that a therapeutic break-through was effected with the production of an anti-bilharzia drug named Miracil D or Nilodin, which could be taken by mouth. Its synthesis was followed by that of a more effective compound named Ambilhar, and today still more potent compounds are available.

Yet far more important than the cure of established disease is its prevention. This enormous problem may be considered under three heads: avoidance of human contact with snails, environmental sanitation, and destruction of snails.

Prevention of human contact with the snail vector can clearly best be achieved by educating those at risk about all elements of the disease and the ways of avoiding infection (which indeed may be impossible if the people are engaged in growing rice). In addition, human exposure to bilharzia would be drastically reduced by the provision of piped supplies of water and safe washing facilities in every village, while environmental sanitation would be ensured through the proper disposal of excreta in simple domestic latrines of the deep pit type. Other innovations are helpful in fighting bilharzia, such as the lining of irrigation furrows with cement which discourages snails, the intermittent irrigation of paddy fields since this appears to upset the parasite's life cycle, and storage of water away from snails for two or three days which exceeds the survival time of the cercariae.

Widespread destruction of snails, however, appeared to offer the easiest way of dealing with the bilharzia problem in tropical Africa, and a great deal of work in this field has been accomplished. Leiper was the first to suggest the addition of ammonium sulphate as a molluscicide to infested water. Copper sulphate was subsequently found to be more lethal to snails, and in its natural form, malachite, was reasonably cheap to apply.

Molluscicides, however, possess certain disadvantages; for one thing they are not all poisonous to snail eggs which are anyway extremely difficult to identify, and they are expensive when used on a large scale. Accordingly, a wide search was made for naturally occurring snail poisons which would be cheaper and more effective than chemical molluscicides. At Nkhotakota we carried out experiments with many substances which persuaded us that a wild perennial shrub named *Tephrosia vogelii* was eminently suitable for the purpose. Growing abundantly beside lakeside pools, the shrub reaches a height of two metres, and enough was available to deal with all local snail breeding grounds in the town's vicinity. Harmless to man, it was used by the Africans as a fish poison and it proved equally effective in killing snails. Pleas to initiate bilharzia control by means of this naturally occurring shrub were, however, frowned upon by the dead hand of colonial authority, and resulted only in my transfer to the highlands of Malawi where very little bilharzia occurred. But research into the use of natural snail poisons continues, and it is interesting to note that another common weed, *Ambrosia maritima*, has recently been recommended as a molluscicide in Egypt.

Biological control of snails has also been attempted through the introduction of snail-eating fish into bilharzial water, but again application of this method on a large scale would be ruinously expensive. Even more costly would be the suggested introduction into Africa of a snail from Puerto

Rico named *Marisa cornuarietis* which is said to feed on the eggs of other snails. However promising some of these methods may appear, no molluscicide is likely to be entirely effective. For snails mature when only two months old and at once begin repeatedly laying clutches of eggs numbering between twenty and thirty. Theoretically it is possible for a single pair of snails which have survived application of poison to rebuild a colony of three million snails within a year.

Most of the suggested methods of control then carry with them the taint of impracticability, and the hopes of tropical Africa today with respect to bilharzia are pinned on the work of sanitary engineers and the production of a vaccine which will protect its people against infection and damage by the fluke's eggs. The search for a vaccine promises good results and it will be diligently pursued. For every year that passes only serves to enlarge the bilharzial empire in Central Africa, and the infirmity it causes remains one of the continent's most weighty problems.

11

The Lesser Terrors
of Kachindomoto

THIS CHAPTER HAS been devoted to what I have termed the 'lesser terrors' of the village which for me had come to symbolise the very essence of Africa, its beauty and its ugliness. But there was nothing minor about the effects of these 'lesser' infections. Though not usually so lethal as those conditions already considered, they added grievously to the burden of disease carried by the African peoples, reduced their productivity and helped to perpetuate the socio--economic inertia which so influenced the destiny of sub-Saharan Africa.

*   *   *

Without doubt the most common infection was the mystifying affliction which we called tropical ulcer. In other parts of the world it was also known as Yemen ulcer, Naga sore, Cochin sore, and a dozen other names which proclaimed its wide distribution through the tropics and our ignorance of its cause.

All the doctors stationed on the lake shore of Malawi spent a great deal of their time treating these ulcers, and the monthly reports to Headquarters continually described promising results obtained by a variety of new and sometimes bizarre methods. In fact, the only course that seemed at all effective was admission to hospital where the patients would be sure of obtaining a more nutritious diet than their usual fare in the bush.

Children and young men were most often affected by tropical ulcers. They would line up outside hospitals and dispensaries, each displaying a chronic ulcer and ruefully

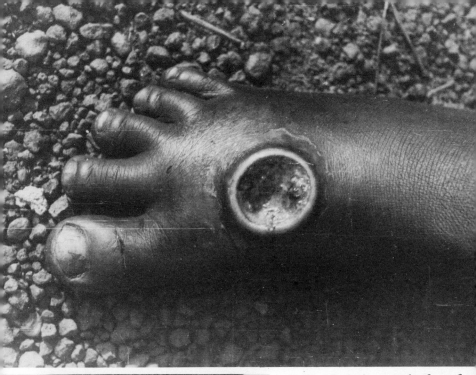

8 Tropical ulcer on the foot of an African patient before treatment

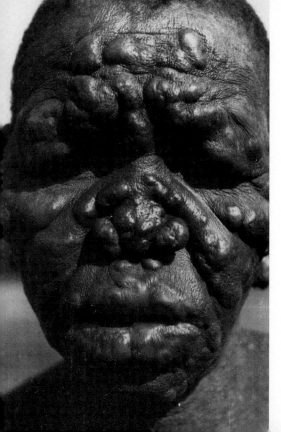

9 Advanced leprosy in an African patient

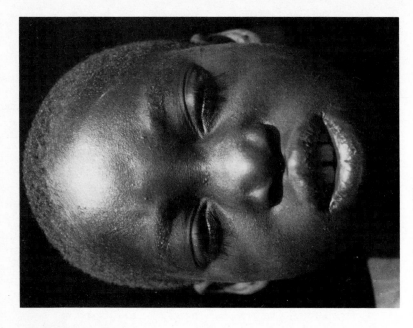

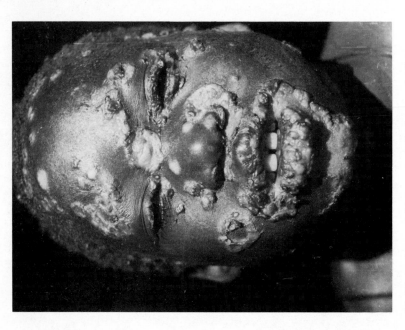

10 Yaws in an African youth before and after treatment with long-acting penicillin

comparing its size with those of their friends. Most of the ulcers occurred on the shin or foot. If neglected they would penetrate so deeply as to expose the tendons of the limb, and even eat into the bones.

David Hunter, an early practitioner in Jamaica, seems to have been the first man to refer to these gangrenous ulcers. In 1792 he described them very well: 'the sores,' he wrote, 'spread quickly, and form large ulcerated surfaces. The granulations turn flaccid and even mortify in parts. The portion skinned over mortifies afresh, and the sore becomes larger than ever. Ulcers of some standing cannot be healed.'

The pain and irritation from these terrible sores would have immobilised most white men, but the Africans bore them with remarkable stoicism, suggesting that their threshold of pain was far higher than that of Europeans. The cause of tropical ulcers was a favourite source of dispute. Certainly a diphtheria-like organism was frequently found in the sores, but it was probably a secondary invader. Indeed, it has been suggested that its prevalence and the immunising effect exerted on the population may account for the relative rarity of diphtheria in equatorial Africa. Usually the ulceration followed some minor injury to the legs, even so slight as a scratch from a thorn or a rubbed mosquito bite. A bleb then formed over the site and ruptured into a spreading, sloughing, fly-blown sore from which oozed stinking yellow pus.

These ulcers are especially associated with famine and war, and members of the Africa Carrier Corps were terribly affected during the 1914–1918 campaign in East Africa. Unfortunately, it was not appreciated at the time that the gangrenous sores were related to chronic malnutrition and especially to protein deficiency.

David Livingstone once suffered from these 'irritable-eating ulcers' for eight months, and only cured himself, after taking advice from Arab slavers, by the application of powdered malachite, and indeed copper sulphate dressings remained a popular treatment for many years. Other commonly used applications included boracic powder, iodoform and arsenic preparations, but all were discarded in turn until the magic qualities of penicillin were recognised.

As always, prevention of these gangrenous ulcers remains more important than their cure. This can be achieved by dressing all abrasions and cuts about the legs with an antibiotic ointment, while the wearing of puttees protects them against minor injury. But the real solution to what once seemed an intractable problem lies in improving the peasants' nutrition with diets rich in first-class protein and vitamins.

*   *   *

Some distance from Kachindomoto stood a remote mission station belonging to the White Fathers. This complex of brick buildings, all battlements and turrets, wore a vaguely teutonic appearance. It looked very substantial beside the mission's neighbouring leper colony where a community of outcasts dragged out their existence. It was well peopled.

About one hundred and twenty leprosy victims together with several billion flies, inhabited this forlorn asylum. Our visits there revealed a scene of indescribable squalor. The mud huts leaned drunkenly together like ricketty toys; their walls were crumbling; the roofs of ancient, greying thatch provided some shelter from the blistering sun but very little from the summer rains. Anguish and antipathy were curiously combined in this corner of an earthly hell. When we appeared for the first time, most of the inmates lay stretched out, motionless on their straw sleeping mats, but a few sat crouched together, engaged in endless, drooling conversation. Then, as the lepers looked up and saw us, the scene changed as though life had been pumped back into the inert figures, and they came stumbling and crawling up to where we stood, stretching out ulcerated begging hands, grinning and grimacing, relieved to see these strangers who had made a break in the grey pattern of their existence. For the rare visitors might care for their misfortune and even be generous with little gifts of food.

All the biblical descriptions and subconscious ancestral memories of leprosy in medieval England stirred in our minds as we watched the approaching, mutilated figures. Many of them had lost their toes and fingers, others whole hands. In some the noses had collapsed into unsightly blobs of flesh and gristle. Most of the inmates also exhibited unhealed burns and sores, partly covered by grimy bandages whose loose ends trailed behind them in the dust. Almost all pointed to plaques of thickened skin which added to the horror of their decayed and rotting faces. A few were blind, their eyes grey with scarring, yet able still to weep.

It was long accepted that leprosy was an infection confined to the human race, but recently animals, including mice, have been artificially infected under laboratory conditions with the causative germ. Leprosy was widespread in Europe during the Middle Ages but today it is confined to the tropics and sub-tropics.

It has been said that leprosy (which comes from the Greek word for 'scaley') is 'as old as the world itself'. The Bible several times refers to the infection, although it is accepted that the signs may have been confused with those of yaws and skin conditions like psoriasis. Ancient papyri speak of the disease in Egypt, and Pompey's troops are reputed to have carried it to Greece and Italy in 62 BC. From there it was disseminated throughout the Roman world with the legions. By the eighth century AD, the malady had become extremely common in Europe and its incidence increased after the crusades. It now began to play a larger part in men's lives than any other malady, especially in their imagination and in their art, as many painters demonstrated when they took pains to include lepers in their canvasses. The cause of the disease was unknown, but generally regarded as a punishment for personal sin or heresy. Edward the Confessor suffered from leprosy but was miraculously cured. Robert the Bruce and King

Baldwin IV of Jerusalem died from it.

So prevalent did leprosy become in Europe during the Middle Ages that both State and Church moved to deal with the crisis. Together they instituted a crude form of quarantine by treating leprosy sufferers as outcasts. They were compelled to wear gloves and distinctive clothing, provided with a bell or clapper to warn of their approach, and ordered to shout 'unclean, unclean' as they moved about. In addition the lepers were forbidden to drink from public fountains, speak loudly, eat with healthy persons, or attend church services, although from outside they might watch the Elevation of the Host through the 'squints' which can still be seen in the old churches of England.

In later years those suffering from leprosy were immured for life in asylums. By 1300 some nineteen thousand lazarettos or leprosaria are known to have existed in Christendom, most of them in France. In some countries the Church pronounced lepers to be legally dead, and held burial services over the living outcasts during which the doleful Mass of St Lazarus was read. In tropical Africa, lepers were simply driven into the forest to die.

Such rigid isolation undoubtedly played a part in ridding Europe of the scourge, but other valid factors have been recognised as assisting in its elimination. Thus it has been noted that feeding habits in Europe changed after the thirteenth century, and vegetables became popular enough to enrich the general diet. In addition, housing and sanitation improved, while clothing became warmer and more sophisticated, especially after the onset of the 'little Ice Age' at the end of the medieval period. It has also been suggested that the Black Death exterminated all lepers and that a rising incidence of tuberculosis conferred some immunity against leprosy whose bacillus is related to that of tuberculosis. Whatever may have been the cause, the ancient scourge abated in Europe and presently the leprosaria stood empty and abandoned. The last indigenous leprosy victim in England died during 1798. The disease dragged on in Scandinavia for another century.

The leprosy we saw in Africa was characterised by slow mutilation of its victims' bodies. Its stigmata usually appeared during childhood and affected twice as many males as females. The disease is caused by a large bacillus which was first reported during 1873 by a Norwegian pathologist named Armauer Hansen, long before the proper establishment of bacteriology as a science. We still do not understand how the leprosy bacillus is transmitted to man, but the course of the disease is well known. Once the leprosy bacilli have entered the body they tend to spread along the nerves to its different parts, though usually sparing warm areas such as the arm-pit. According to their hosts' degree of immunity the disease appears in two different forms, (although intermediate types may be recognised). One is a mild self-limiting disease which is called tuberculoid leprosy; in it the only sign of infection may be minimal bleaching of the skin. The second type appears where the hosts' immunity reactions are less effective, and this is termed lepromatous leprosy. In it, massive destruction of the nerves results in foot-drop, wrist-drop, deformity of the feet and chronic ulceration of the limbs with loss of fingers and toes. In such cases the skin may also become greatly thickened, and this when affecting the face gives to it a curiously leonine appearance. In some lepromatous cases, blindness follows the involvement of the eyes, while when the larynx is affected stridor and obstruction to breathing occur. It is no wonder that the grossly mutilating signs of lepromatous infection made it one of mankind's most dreaded diseases.

The manifestations of leprosy have not altered over the ages. Those seen by a medieval observer in England set him writing about 'the eyebrows falling bare and getting knotted with uneven tuberosities, the nose and other features becoming thick, coarse and lumpy, the face losing its mobility of play of expression, the raucous voice, the loss of sensibility in the hands and the ultimate break-up or maufragium of the leprous growths into foul running sores.' His description fits the signs of the disease today.

The method of spread of leprosy from person to person has been much debated, but contact transmission is strongly suggested by its frequent appearance in several members of a family. Many insect vectors of the germ have been suspected, but are now disproven. Leprosy is not inherited; it only occurs following long contact with the disease, yet strangely it rarely appears in both husband and wife. The majority of people who nursed in leper colonies escaped the disease, but it has still claimed a toll of victims of whom probably Father Damien (1840–89) is the best known.

Leprosy has long been established in Africa. By 1950 an estimated one and a half million lepers were living in the tropical part of the continent. It was particularly common in the Congo, where in some villages half the inhabitants suffered from it. The manifestations of the disease usually appear between the ages of sixteen and twenty.

Few lepers were seen during the early years of European contact, since they had been driven away into the bush perhaps to keep them out of sight, but after the demonstrably good results obtained from western medicine became appreciated, they flocked to administrative centres seeking help. Because of the lurid European experience in the past, much attention was paid to their plight, especially by missionary bodies. Chaulmoogra oil was then the sheet anchor of their therapy. The yellow oil, which smells like rancid butter, is expressed from an evergreen shrub named *Hydnocarpus kurzii* which grows freely in the Far East. Chaulmoogra is a very ancient remedy, much used in China and India, but ignored by European doctors until the middle of the last century. It was usually given by mouth and inunction, but sometimes injected into affected areas of skin. Treatment was necessarily prolonged, and because so many years passed before the course of leprosy could be arrested, many practitioners doubted its efficacy, although the Africans always retained their confidence in this unpleasant therapy.

Then, during the early 1940s, treatment was revolutionised by the introduction of a group of drugs named the sulphones. For the first time in history a truly specific remedy for leprosy had become available. Fortunately it was comparatively cheap, easily obtained and permitted treatment to be given at home; all factors which encouraged its acceptance by the Africans. The sulphones do not cure leprosy, but rather suppress it, so that early treatment is important.

Some of the terrible deformities which once complicated the disease can be treated effectively by physiotherapy and surgery, but prevention of the infection should take precedence over its amelioration. Education about the disease is still an important factor in preventing leprosy, but this must be associated with the raising of the general standard of living in Black Africa and especially by the provision of nutritious food, clean clothing and uncrowded living quarters. Isolation of children from leprous parents must be ensured, and infected persons discouraged from having children, not only for the sake of the babies but also because pregnancy often activates an infection of the disease. But thanks to modern therapy lepers are no longer shunned by their relatives but lead normal lives.

There is now a further prospect of an advance which may ultimately eliminate leprosy from the continent. For years scientists have endeavoured to develop a protective vaccine against the disease, but they failed through lack of living leprosy germs, for it proved impossible to cultivate these bacilli in the laboratory. Recently, however, it was found that the leprosy bacillus multiplies when injected into armadillos. These inoffensive creatures live in the tropical and temperate regions of the Americas. They measure about twelve inches long and are protected by solid buckler-like plates. The armadillo's body temperature is low and probably this factor favours the reproduction of leprosy bacilli. Scientists now possess a rich source of the bacillus and are hopeful of producing a vaccine which will provide total protection against the disease.

*   *   *

A few years ago it seemed likely that Kachindomoto would soon be rid of another of its terrors: the disease called yaws by the British and framboesia by Germans since its skin lesions resemble ripe raspberries.

Yaws is a disease of hot climates which cripples and mutilates its victims rather than kills them. It affects rural populations and was particularly common in tropical Africa. The disease was probably present among hunting, food-gathering human bands who once roamed the continent. In such small communities yaws survived only because patients may suffer relapses for five years or more after they are infected. For many purposes, yaws may be regarded as a latent infection with relapses of active disease.

Essentially yaws is a skin disease which forms deep, open sores all over the body. Infection usually occurs at about the age of three when a child's movements extend beyond the family range. Until recently a high proportion of Africans were infected by yaws by the age of fifteen. Infection after thirty is rare.

The initial yaws lesion appears commonly on the skin of the lower leg. It is raspberry-like in appearance. Some three months later the eruption becomes generalised. The raised sores exude a clear fluid, teeming with infective organisms. The exudate dries to form yellow crusts. This wide-spread eruption heals by itself after a few months but may relapse within a year, and again heal. This may be repeated several times in the first five years of the disease. These changes are not destructive and on healing leave little or no scarring.

There is then a period of five or ten years or more when there may be no sign of the disease. This quiescent period is followed by further relapses of active disease, but now destructive skin and bone changes occur, and on healing some six months later, they leave scars. These scars on the skin may contract and tie up elbows and knees. Thickening of the palms and soles occurs and may restrict the use of hands and feet, and thus interfere with essential agricultural work. Pain in bones may be prominent at all stages. Yaws is a crippling disease; indeed during the 1940s, in parts of the Congo, it was considered to be a greater burden on the people than all the other diseases from which they suffered. Serological surveys suggest that infection rates of yaws in parts of Middle Africa at that time were over eighty per cent.

During 1905, while working in Ceylon, Sir Aldo Castellani, hero of the great sleeping sickness debate, identified the causal organism of yaws as a twisted organism which he found swarming in the sores of infected patients. These spirochaetes or treponemes are minute threadlike, spiral organisms, and because they are actively motile some authorities regard them as belonging to the animal world. The spirochaete of yaws, named *Treponema pertenue*, is physically indistinguishable from the organisms causing syphilis, and childhood infection with yaws protects the patient against this dreaded venereal disease of adults.

Bones dating from AD 850 have been found with typical yaws lesions, and during the tenth century Arab physicians wrote clear descriptions of its manifestations in Africa. Fifteenth-century Portuguese reported yaws as being prevalent among the inhabitants of tropical Africa. The disease became common on slave ships and was thus carried to the New World.

No evidence of insect transmission of yaws has ever been proved, and the infection is almost certainly transferred by direct bodily contact, usually in childhood and often on fingers soiled by serum from an infected sore which then infect minor abrasions on a healthy person's skin. The Africans accept it as a contagious disease.

African methods of treatment varied; two favoured 'cures' were the application of lime paste and blacksmith's rubbish to the sores. At first European therapy was scarcely more effective: it was based on prescribing mercury salts by mouth, a treatment credited to Sir Thomas Sydenham who wrote of his intention to 'carry off [yaws] with a salivation raised by quicksilver'.

After the First World War the introduction of the injection of bismuth and arsenic drugs as a treatment brought about a notable decrease of the disease. Their effectiveness made a deep impression on the natives of tropical Africa, and a Scots medical missionary in 1925 was certain that 'it was the injection treatment for yaws which firmly established the success of [European] medical work . . . and brought the people in hitherto unimagined numbers about the doors of the hospitals.' He went on to note that 'scarcely a child escaped the contagious yaws infection [in Southern Nigeria] which spreads in unsightly and painful sores over the face and throughout the body until there is hardly a clean inch of skin to be seen. There is no more pitiful sight in Africa than a child scaled from head to foot by the broken sores of yaws and tormented by the flies which settle on each festering patch. Later in life the disease returns in the shape of twisted limbs, swollen feet and wracking pains in bones, bringing misery with the chill rains of every wet season.'

The Scots doctor was perfectly correct in ascribing the Africans' increasing trust in western medicine to the dramatic effects on yaws of bismuth salts (given intramuscularly) and arsenic compounds (used intravenously). After their introduction the sufferers came crowding up for treatment with the magic needle which they called the 'sewing machine'.

The fall in the prevalence of yaws in Africa which followed the use of these drugs may have impressed the Africans, but a far more dramatic decrease resulted from the subsequent introduction of long-acting penicillin (PAM). With assistance from the World Health Organisation (WHO) and the United Nations International Children's Fund (UNICEF), mass campaigns were undertaken in endemic areas of Africa. PAM was given to entire communities; this cured florid yaws and suppressed the far

more numerous latent infections. The results were gratifying. Thus in Tanganyika, where earlier surveys had
shown a ninety per cent prevalence of yaws, by 1948 only
fifty thousand cases from the whole territory were notified
and ten years later, after the use of PAM, the infection was
virtually eliminated. Similar results were obtained in all
parts of the sub-continent. Not all the credit for this should
be ascribed to the new drugs; some may have been due to
a rising standard of living in black communities, to the
growing use of soap which may prevent infective organisms
from penetrating the skin, and the increasing wearing of
clothing which protects the skin from infectious contact.

Unfortunately, the PAM campaigns were not always followed up. It had been intended that, from rural health
centres in the freed areas, staff would treat new cases of
yaws and their contacts; lack of funds or of suitable staff did
not always allow the establishment of this essential surveillance, and the eradication of yaws from Africa has been
delayed. A cause of great concern, however, is the exposure
of a rising generation of Africans, which for twenty years
or more has now been free from yaws, to infection with
syphilis. For the incidence of syphilis is rising today in Black
Africa, and the cause may largely be the loss of immunity to
the disease previously gained by childhood infection with
yaws.

This trend has induced protracted argument among
scientific circles about the relationship between yaws and
its near relative, syphilis. The two infections share many
features: the causal spirochaetes are identical in appearance, both provide cross immunity so that infection with one
protects against the other, and they respond to the same
therapy treatment.

Yet for all these shared properties the infections produce
very different symptoms. Yaws affects man's skin and
bones; syphilis attacks all human tissue and is particularly
damaging to heart muscle, the nervous system (causing
paralysis and insanity), and the placenta (which may result

in congenital syphilis). There is good evidence too that yaws is a much older disease than syphilis, as is shown by its presence in skeletons dating back a thousand years, whereas syphilis as we know it, only made its appearance towards the end of the fifteenth century. Then again, yaws is a non-venereal disease, being transmitted through skin contact between children, whereas syphilis is generally transferred during coitus to the mucous membranes of the sexual organs and sometimes of the mouth. Moreover, yaws is an infection of peasant communities while syphilis wins its greatest victories in urban areas and affects all social classes.

Many theories have been advanced to explain the differences and similarities of the two diseases. Thus it has been suggested that they are caused by two different strains of the same organism, or that the quality of a common spirochaete alters in differing climatic conditions. The latter theory is supported by the occurrence of another disease caused by a spirochaete which in appearance is identical to those of syphilis and yaws. This infection, treponarid (endemic syphilis), occurs in hot dry countries on both sides of the warm tropical belt in Africa, being seen in countries like Niger and Botswana. The properties of its spirochaete are intermediate between those of yaws and syphilis, suggesting an adaptation – perhaps eight to ten thousand years ago – to allow its survival in changing climatic conditions.

It seems possible to suggest that Negro slaves carried yaws to Europe during the fifteenth century, and there its causal organism, seeking like all parasites to increase its empire, found a temperate climate inimical to its ambitions. For skin to skin transmission was difficult when prospective hosts were well clad and in the process of improving their personal hygiene. Instead of continuing to live in running sores, the spirochaetes of yaws supposedly then found a means of infecting the mucous membranes of the human sexual organs. In other words it altered in such a way as to develop the capacity for venereal transmission and the ability to attack human tissues other than the skin. It now found a multitude of human hosts in Europe which, having been long free from yaws, presented no resistance to this new germ. But this is pure conjecture, and no scientific facts can be put forward to sustain it.

Advocates of the theory support it by pointing out that syphilis made its first appearance, and in florid form, only towards the end of the fifteenth century. It broke out then among the troops of Charles VIII of France when they were laying siege to Naples, affecting them so acutely as to suggest that resistance to it was minimal, and that this therefore was a new human disease. When the siege was raised the soldiers and camp followers spread the previously unknown infection throughout Europe. Contemporary Frenchmen called it the 'English disease' while the English returned the compliment by naming it the 'French disease', and they believed it was spread in the breath. Among the accusations laid against Cardinal Wolsey was one of passing syphilis on to Henry VIII (who was clearly infected) while 'whispering in his ear', and indeed the Tudor method of greeting each other by kissing may have been a factor in disseminating the disease in England.

During the sixteenth century the symptoms of syphilis became milder due to mutual adjustments between host and parasite which led to less severe clinical manifestations and a higher survival rate for the spirochaete. The lowered incidence of florid syphilis was noted as early as 1529 by Sir Thomas More in his book *Supplycacyon of Soulys*, and confirmed fifty years later by the surgeon William Clowes.

Most authorities have now abandoned the popular notion that syphilis originated in the New World and was brought back to Europe by Columbus's mariners. For one thing, a treponemal disease named pinta was present in America before 1492, and this infection, like yaws, protects against syphilis. Nor does it seem likely that Columbus's returning sailors, who numbered less than fifty, could have passed on the spirochaete so effectively that within eighteen months it had spread through the whole of Europe.

No doubt syphilis was brought to tropical Africa by the slave trade, but it does not appear to have spread inland for some time. Livingstone found no evidence of the disease during his extensive travels in the interior between 1840 and his death thirty-three years later. By 1900, however, syphilis was occurring in East Africa. Albert Cook in Uganda even stated that venereal disease came to be the most important part of his work, and another missionary claimed that 'the immense majority [of his patients] have fallen ill through immorality'. The dramatic increase in venereal disease suggests that the Arab traders entering Africa from the east were partly responsible for the introduction of both syphilis and gonorrhoea.

Yaws was a terrible burden for the inhabitants of old Africa, but at least the infection appears to have protected them, through cross-immunity, from the more serious effects of syphilis. Today the situation has altered. The incidence of yaws has dropped and the protection it previously provided against syphilis is fading. And as syphilis increases in the continent it is feared that fulminating infections of this disease may begin to make their appearance in a replay of the terrible epidemic which affected Europe nearly five hundred years ago.

　　　　*　　　　　　*　　　　　　*

Jigger fleas were a curse to the people living on the lakeshore of Nyasa. The fleas' original home was Brazil, and they were introduced into West Africa during 1872 by the infested crew of a British ship, *Thomas Mitchell*. They spread rapidly across the continent in company with sleeping sickness, many of the fleas travelling part of the way in the ballast of Congo steamships. The fleas reached the east coast of Africa by 1895; three years later they were in Zanzibar and soon afterwards appeared in Bombay and Karachi.

The adult fleas measure about one millimetre in length

and live in sandy soil which they leave periodically to suck the blood of warm-blooded animals including man. When impregnated, the female flea burrows into the skin between man's toes and under the toe nails. There the flea swells up to the size of a small pea causing intense irritation; its back end lies in the opening of the skin, and through it numerous eggs are passed. Finally, the flea is expelled, leaving a small ulcer behind which is likely to become septic. The infection is liable to spread and lead to the destruction of toes and even of the legs. Members of Emin Pasha's expedition saw people on the shores of Lake Victoria whose entire legs had rotted off; their villages were deserted and the fields unharvested. In Angola sepsis following jigger infection became only second to smallpox as a cause of death during the decades which followed the fleas' introduction to Africa.

During 1897 Lord Baden-Powell was badly affected by jigger fleas while campaigning in Southern Rhodesia. 'Curious,' he wrote, 'how the little pest should be able to cross Africa and make himself a scourge in a new bit of Africa . . . taking only three years to get here from Somaliland.' Africans are skilled at removing the fleas with needles, and they brought much relief to several generations of European expatriates. Modern hygiene has greatly curbed this, one of the minor but sometimes dangerous, scourges of tropical Africa. It is said that the irritation caused by these fleas gave rise to the phrase 'I'll be jiggered'.

*   *   *

The bloody flux was another common cause of illness in sub-Saharan Africa and seen frequently at Kachindomoto. The condition results from inflammation of the lower part of the intestine. It is now usually called dysentery, a name derived from the Greek and meaning 'bowel trouble'.

Dysentery was well known in ancient Egypt, one of whose gods, Osiris, is supposed to have suffered from it. It killed both Edward I and his son, the Black Prince, whose untimely death led to the early succession of Richard II and ultimately to the disastrous Wars of the Roses. Dysentery may be divided into two main groups: one is due to an animal parasite of man named *Entamoeba histolytica*; the other type is caused by a bacillus.

Amoebic dysentery occurs all over the world but is most prevalent in the tropics and probably accounts for the majority of bloody flux in the sub-Saharan Africa. In some parts of West Africa, nearly half the inhabitants harbour the responsible parasite.

These parasites are single-celled organisms belonging to the animal kingdom which normally live as commensals in the human gut. They are too primitive to have acquired the advantages and handicaps of sexuality, and multiply simply by dividing into two. The amoebae are microscopic in size, measuring about one thousandth of a millimetre. Under the microscope they look like blobs of jelly which constantly change their shape. They feed peacefully by ingestion of bacteria and waste material in the lower gut of their human hosts, but they are treacherous, capricious organisms. Suddenly, for some reason as yet not understood, they turn from commensalism and invade the intestinal wall, producing ulceration which is manifest by bloody diarrhoea.

To survive as a species the parasite must get its progeny out of the host's body, and the one possible exit is through the anus with the faeces. To remain alive they must next be swallowed by a new human host. This occurs when food has been contaminated by flies or through the eating of vegetables that have been manured. The parasite will now face the problem of passing safely through the acid digestive juice in its new host's stomach before it reaches its final goal, his lower bowel.

Some survive this challenge by building protective shells around themselves, the tiny blobs of jelly turning into spherical cysts. These pass unscathed when swallowed but when they reach the lower bowel their walls are dissolved by an intestinal ferment named trypsin. This releases the imprisoned protozoa which divide into four small amoebae and so continue the cycle.

Severe amoebiasis in man may be a very acute disease whereby the patient suffers from repeated passage of bloody stools. But more usually he experiences chronic sickness with mild diarrhoea, loss of weight, dyspepsia and anaemia. Occasionally the protozoa enter the host's blood stream and are carried to the liver where they form abscesses which if not diagnosed and treated may be fatal.

Because of similar symptoms, amoebiasis was long confused with bacillary dysentery, and it was not until 1870 that Timothy Lewis reported the presence of amoebic protozoa in the faeces of a dysenteric patient. Five years later a Russian, E. Lösch, found this same organism in the stools of a peasant named Markoff who subsequently died of the infection. Before his death Lösch fed Markoff's stools to a dog, which soon passed cysts in its faeces.

This work allowed scientists to divide the dysenteries into two main groups: an endemic illness due to amoebae and an epidemic flux named bacillary dysentery since it was caused by a bacillus.

By 1891 exact descriptions had been written of the causal organism of amoebic dysentery, but its association with liver abscesses was not appreciated for some years. Even Manson erred by insisting that these dangerous abscesses in the liver resulted from an unwise intake of food and alcohol by Europeans in the tropics.

During the First World War many soldiers went down with amoebic dysentery and this initiated fresh research into the disease. E.L. Walker and A.W. Sellards were the first to feed amoebic cysts to twenty human volunteers; eighteen promptly went down with amoebiasis, and the life cycle of the parasite was finally confirmed.

A preparation of the dried roots of the *Cephaëlis ipecacuanha* plant, a native of Brazil and the Far East, was well known since ancient times as a cure for dysentery. Sir Leonard Rogers now proceeded to isolate one of its alkaloids, emetine. He prescribed this with excellent results in acute amoebiasis, and it became the accepted treatment for the infection. Emetine had no effect, however, on bacillary dysentery. Prevention of infection with amoebae is obtained basically by the protection of food from flies, and the avoidance of contaminated water and uncooked vegetables.

Bacillary dysentery causes symptoms very similar to those of amoebiasis. It occurs in temperate climates but is most commonly seen in the tropics. Essentially it is a fly-borne disease to which adult Africans have developed a fair degree of immunity, but infants are highly susceptible. The bacillus does not undergo development within flies; it is simply transferred on their soiled legs to footstuffs.

Of ancient origin the infection is mentioned in Egyptian papyri from 1600 BC, but it was not distinguished from its amoebic counterpart until 1898 when a Japanese scientist named Shiga isolated the causative bacillus. Its symptoms vary from mild diarrhoea to fulminating symptoms where the patient passes as many as fifty stools a day consisting almost entirely of mucus and blood. Fortunately, in the sulphonamides we now possess an effective drug for the infection, while great advances have been made in the restoration of lost fluid and salt by intravenous replacement. The lives of many children suffering from dysentery and other diarrhoeal diseases are saved every day by 'drip therapy', but unfortunately this requires treatment in a well-equipped hospital under physicians' supervision.

For ten years the scientists of the World Health Organisation grappled with the problem of providing fluid replacement to people living in rural areas which lacked hospital facilities. They eventually discovered that ninety-five per cent of children suffering from diarrhoea would respond to swallowing thirty millilitres (about one ounce) of fluid, fortified with salts, at fifteen minute intervals (if larger quantities are given at one time they cause vomiting). The recommended formula is made up of sodium chloride (common salt) 3.5 gram, potassium chloride 2.5 gram, and glucose 20 gram in one litre of potable water.

Equipped with sulphonamide tablets and packages of these ingredients for solution, primary care staff can now treat most of the infants suffering from dysentery, and only five per cent will require hospitalisation. The danger from one more hazard of Africa has thus been notably lessened.

As with amoebiasis, prevention of dysentery is essentially a problem of fly control. The provision of adequate sanitary equipment and proper protection of food must be achieved before the dysenteries are finally banished from the continent.

*   *   *

Yet another serious problem at Kachindomoto, and indeed throughout East and Central Africa, was relapsing fever which, after malaria, sleeping sickness and bilharzia, may become the fourth most widespread disease in the continent, and one whose domain has been greatly facilitated by improved communications.

David Livingstone was the first person to record the existence of relapsing fever and its method of transmission. During the May of 1854, while on the first leg of his famous trans-African journey, he stayed at the Portuguese station of Ambaca, some two hundred and fifty kilometres east of Luanda. In his book *Missionary Travels* he noted that he had been bitten by a tick about the size of a pin's head and which was to be found in all the local mud huts. He went on to write that this tick sucks human blood 'until quite full' and that if the patient does not vomit 'fever sets in; and I was assured by an intelligent Portuguese there that death has sometimes been the result of this fever.' Livingstone further remarked that his African porters recognised and had 'cause to dread this insignificant insect' as the carrier of a fever. Some two years later while at Tete he again turned his attention to this tick-borne disease, remarking that in curing the bite of the tampan, the natives administer 'one of the insects . . . in the medicine employed'.

Relapsing fever occurs all over Africa today as well as in many other parts of the world. It is said to have originated from a focus in the lower Zambezi valley. There perhaps we can imagine a strain of free-living ticks which had grown weary of the everlasting chore of seeking out suitable decaying vegetable matter to eat. Either through innate intelligence or perhaps through fortuitous contact with human blood, they found that they could obtain food more easily by attaching themselves to a human host. For this benefactor would provide them with a generous supply of rich red nourishment from only periodic bites. While feeding an infected tick would pass on the spirochaete of relapsing fever.

From the Zambezi, relapsing fever spread across the continent to the Atlantic seaboard, its migration being in the opposite direction to that of sleeping sickness and the jigger flea. It was recognised in Zaire during 1903 by a British medical team which had come out to investigate sleeping sickness at the invitation of the Belgian government. The members of this team were J. Everett Dutton, Cuthbert Christy and John Todd, the first two we have already met among the early workers with sleeping sickness.

After taking note of the high incidence of relapsing fever among the local Africans, this team began to investigate the infection. The Africans were well aware of a tick's association with the disease, and Dutton and his co-workers were quickly able to identify it as *Ornithodorus moubata*. The team went on to incriminate a blood spirochaete as the causal organism. Unfortunately both Dutton and Todd became infected during their investigations and Dutton died before their discoveries were made known.

When tropical Africa was in the grip of famine during the period 1915–25, sleeping sickness, influenza, smallpox, meningitis, and also relapsing fever became widespread. The latter's symptoms were similar to those of malaria except that the bouts of fever were repeated at regular intervals despite quinine therapy. Today relapsing fever is in a quiescent period and its mortality is low.

The *Ornithodorus* tick which Dutton and his colleagues identified as the vector of the disease, can only move about thirty yards on its own, and it relies on man and other animal hosts for further transport. It seeks to live in human dwellings particularly in places such as rest houses, schools and prisons where the population is constantly changing. In these the insects make their homes in cracks and crevices of the walls and floors, venturing out at night to feed on the sleeping human inmates.

The precise method of transmission of relapsing fever spirochaetes by the tick remains unknown. Probably the tick passes on the organisms when biting, but the spirochaetes may be deposited in the insect's faeces and then be rubbed into the itching bite-wound by the human victim.

Africans develop a high degree of immunity to relapsing fever in their own locality, but when they move away, even to a nearby village, they are prone to develop the disease, caused by an unfamiliar strain of the spirochaete against which they have no built-in protection. Such lack of immunity to a local parasite strain was dramatically illustrated in 1962 by the entomologist G.F. Walton. He described the deaths from relapsing fever of a party of Masai tribesmen after they had been imprisoned for a trifling offence in an infected jail at Mwanza, Tanganyika. Walton bitterly commented that 'A three-month prison sentence could be three months rest with free food for the local tick-infested Sukuma tribesmen and a sentence of death for the tick-free Masai who have no immunity to the disease.' The tragic deaths of these Masai, far from their homes beyond Kilimanjaro, haunts me still.

I met Africans in Nyasaland who, when they travelled from their villages, carried a few ticks from their huts in a little box. These they periodically released and allowed the ticks to bite them, thus reinforcing an immunity which was evidently of short duration.

As with yaws and syphilis, injections of arsenical preparations were used in the treatment of relapsing fever until superceded by penicillin. Prevention is largely a matter of destroying ticks with insecticides of which benzene hydrochloride is the most effective, and the provision of well constructed dwellings which deny them suitable habitats.

In some parts of the world including tropical Africa, the spirochaete of relapsing fever is also transmitted to man by lice but it is the tick-borne infection which is the more serious problem in Africa.

*   *   *

Many people in Kachindomoto were blinded by the eye infection, trachoma. It can be claimed that this disease has caused more suffering and economic loss to the world than any other human affliction. It is still one of mankind's most prevalent diseases and is certainly the most frequent cause of blindness. It has been estimated that more than five hundred million people today suffer from trachoma, and of this number about six million are totally blind. In Black Africa, some thirty million people are affected.

Trachoma was well known to the Romans who called it 'trachy', a word derived from the Greek meaning 'roughening' because of its effect on the inner surface of the eyelids. Paul of Tarsus, Cicero, Horace and Pliny all suffered from the infection. The Romans treated it with copper sulphate drops, a remedy which remained in use until recent times. Trachoma was very common in the Middle East and the crusaders carried it to Europe together with leprosy and several other diseases. St Francis of Assisi, when returning from Egypt, contracted a severe infection and was almost totally blind when he died. It became common among the underprivileged in England, and Moorfields Hospital in London was founded to deal with it.

Bonaparte's army in Egypt suffered severely from trachoma, and also the soldiers of the British expeditionary force which finally expelled the French. Out of the seven hundred men in one English battalion, six hundred and thirty-five were infected by trachoma, of whom fifty lost the sight of both eyes while forty were blinded in one eye. The British government was so shocked by this that it provided pensions for the blind soldiers, the first service pension to be granted.

Today trachoma remains a disease of poverty and over-crowding. Its incidence is related to a shortage of protein intake and an abundance of dust, dirt and flies. In Africa it is essentially a disease of children and particularly of girls who tend to receive less care than boys.

The infection is caused by a virus-like organism and spread in tears, by soiled clothing or towels, and by flies. It is a chronic inflammation of the eye behind the upper eyelid. This tends to turn the eyelids inward so that the lashes cause constant irritation to the eye. The damage extends to the transparent part of the eye producing scarring and diminished vision. In Africa about twenty per cent of the sufferers end up totally blind.

Fortunately, treatment of trachoma is highly effective. Application of an antibiotic ointment to the eye quickly heals early cases, especially if sulphonamides or antibiotics are given orally at the same time. Even a severe case may be cured at a cost of no more than the price of a packet of cigarettes, and mass treatment can be effectively carried out by trained villagers. The irritation of the eye in established cases can be greatly relieved by surgical procedures which lift up the prolapsed lashes. These are carried out by trained doctors.

The incidence of trachoma is now receding before the tide of world civilisation, yet in Middle Africa the area affected is increasing because of continuing low standards of hygiene. It has been said that a small rise in living standards is followed by a large fall in trachoma in a community. Accordingly, if piped water could be provided for every village of Black Africa and a bottle of simple eye drops kept in every dwelling, this bane could be eliminated within a generation. Eradication of trachoma lies within reach; its continued presence on the continent must be regarded as one of the greatest challenges to medical services.

*   *   *

At least the villagers of Kachindomoto were fortunate in being free from an even more terrible hazard to eyesight, a disease named onchocerciasis or river blindness. It occurs in a part of Africa lying between two parameters: one line joins Senegal to Ethiopia, the other stretches from Angola to Tanzania. Onchocerciasis is particularly common in Benin, Ghana, Ivory Coast, Mali, Togo, Niger and Upper Volta. It also occurs in Central America, allegedly carried there from Africa by slave ships, although the French troops of the Emperor Maximilian of Mexico have also been held responsible.

The animal parasite which causes this terrible infection belongs to the same family as the blood fluke which Manson identified as the cause of elephantiasis. The adult worms live in pairs under the human skin and are transmitted to man by a small, black, hump-backed fly, aptly named *Simulium damnosum*. The infection carries a high risk of blindness.

The figures of those infected are among the most daunting in African medicine. Surveys of thirty years ago indicate that between ten and twenty million Africans suffered from onchocerciasis, and that an estimated three million had become completely blind. In some villages thirty per cent of adult men had been blinded by it, and even if you lived in a less infected area one out of every ten of your friends would be sightless.

In Ghana most cases of river blindness occurred among the ten million people living in the upper Volta basin. Of this number an estimated one million suffered from onchocerciasis and seventy thousand were 'economically blind'. Ferrymen, who worked in close contact with the fly transmitters, could look forward to a working expectancy of no more than two years before they were banished to spend the remainder of their lives in darkness. One group of people living in an endemic region of Ghana were so accustomed to blindness that they found difficulty in believing that the rest of the human race could see.

And yet medical men, British, French, Belgian and Portuguese, took an unconscionable time to recognise the heavy toll of human misery caused by river blindness. This was all the more extraordinary since the Africans had long been aware of the association of blindness with lumpy nodules on the sufferers' skin, and with residence near fast-flowing streams. Moreover, the skin lesions of onchocerciasis had been described as long before as 1875 and the responsible parasite identified in 1893. Yet it was only during the 1920s that doctors in Ghana began to associate skin tumours with blindness and Dr D.B. Blacklock of the Liverpool School of Tropical Medicine in 1926 demonstrated the complete life cycle of *Onchocercus volvulus*. Even so the recognition of the havoc it causes was delayed for a further decade. Then during 1936 Mr J.K.G. Syme, the energetic District Commissioner at Bawku in Ghana, informed his headquarters that he had found nine blind men out of two hundred and thirty-two during a routine examination, and that in a neighbouring area five per cent of the men due for hut tax were sightless. Subsequently, in 1944, Dr Harold Ridley reported that a high proportion of Africans at his station of Funsi had nodules of the skin, and of these a third complained of dimness of vision. Four years later Dr B.B. Waddy working near the Volta river, found that nearly ten per cent of local villagers suffered some loss of sight, and noted that the area swarmed with black fly. The people of this region, wrote Waddy, were 'gradually fading out in disease and semi-starvation. . . . The blind are led out to hoe in the fields.' The critical situation had at last been recognised.

The adult female worms which cause river blindness measure up to fifty centimetres in length, while the males are about one tenth as long. Living under the skin, they become twisted together in tangled masses which project as sizeable nodules. They survive there for as long as fifteen years, during which time each female is every year capable of producing about a million filarial larvae. This progeny moves about under the host's skin in the vicinity of the mother nodule, causing intense irritation, particularly when they affect the sole of the foot where it may become so intolerable as to lead to suicide. Some of the microfilariae, especially those from nodules in the patient's head, tend to move into the eye tissues, causing inflammation and eventual blindness. It is these microfilariae which are taken up by black flies when they feed on man.

The Africans in endemic areas long ago learned to avoid living near fast-flowing streams, and many fertile valleys were in consequence abandoned for less promising land beyond the two hundred-kilometre flight range of black fly. They also learned to treat onchocerciasis by excision of the infection's tell-tale nodules, an operation which if repeated often enough will significantly reduce the severity of the individual's infection by simple physical removal of the parasites, the source of the larvae.

The introduction of a new drug named suramin during the 1950s was far more effective but gave rise to dangerous side-effects, and it can only be given under strict medical control. Accordingly, prevention of river blindness is much more important than its treatment. The wearing of adequate clothes provides some protection, and it has been found that a high intake of vitamin A may limit the infection. But it is the destruction of fly breeding places that offers real hope of eliminating this disease, although it is estimated that it will take twenty years to achieve this. The World Health Organisation organised a campaign in 1973 in which five Canadian pilots were stationed in successive affected areas. Piloting helicopters, they hover over the breeding places in fast-running streams that have been identified by ground teams, and spray them with abate which is the most effective insecticide against the larvae.

The control programme extends over most of the countries already mentioned as being most affected, an indication of the importance of not allowing national frontiers to frustrate action against disease. The results have been encouraging: no new cases of onchocerciasis in children under five have been reported since spraying was introduced. Onchocersiasis has also been effectively eliminated in Kenya by spraying and much reduced in Nigeria. Soon, it is hoped, all Africa will be freed from the 'scourge of the river'.

*   *   *

A third African disease due to a member of the filaria family may be briefly considered – guinea worm infestation. Its symptoms are caused by the large female worm, measuring about a metre in length, which wanders about under the human skin in the lower part of the body. When the fertilised worm is ready to eject its larvae, it raises a painful blister on the skin of the host's leg. The blister presently bursts and the worm passes microscopic larvae through the break in the skin when the leg is in water. While in this state the mother worm can be ligatured or lassooed and slowly extracted, an operation which has been practised since earliest times. The male worm is inconsiderable in size and causes no symptoms.

The guinea worm was the first animal parasite of man to be recognised: they were the 'fiery serpents' which tormented the ancient Israelites as narrated in Numbers XXI. Both Plutarch and Galen left accounts of the infection. The life cycle of the worm was discovered as early as 1870, and its transmission by the water flea demonstrated. Man is infected by drinking water containing this intermediate host of the parasite. Thus infection is most likely in the dry season when shrunken water holes concentrate the infected water fleas. The ingested worms would appear on the leg about a year later.

The guinea worm enjoys another more dubious claim to

distinction; the only certain available cure, that of manual removal, has not changed since the days of the Bible, although traditional healers in Africa claim that their herbal remedies cause ejection of the worms. The herbs they recommend are *Combretum mucronatum, Elaeophorbia drupifera*, and *Hilleria latifolia*.

12

The Visitations

IN ADDITION TO the diseases already covered there were the visitations, epidemics that periodically swept through tropical Africa, and were sometimes totally unfamiliar to new generations of its inhabitants. Inevitably, with no immunity, their unwelcome appearances led to a high mortality and also to widespread accusations of sorcery. Sorcery differs from witchcraft in the African mind. In the latter the human agent is deemed unaware of responsibility for any harm inflicted. Sorcery was more feared; it was believed to be practised by ill-intentioned persons who deliberately cast the spells that were responsible for disasters such as famine or outbreaks of enigmatic pestilences like cholera and plague. These epidemics may have appeared erratically but they were particularly demoralising, and greatly reinforced the Africans' helpless acceptance of the inevitability of disease against which there was no remedy and no escape. They included infections imported by Europeans – tuberculosis, measles, whooping cough and the common cold, but potentially the most threatening of them all were the visitations of plague which affected tropical Africa during the past century; fortunately they were rare and of modest extent. Plague is primarily a disease of field rodents, but occasionally the germ affects rats from which it may be transmitted to human beings by fleas. Man, then, enters accidentally into an aberrant cycle of the plague bacillus when the usual rodent-flea-rodent cycle is replaced by a rat-flea-man sequence, after which the germ survives for a period by being passed on through a succession of human hosts.

Perhaps somewhat unfairly, rats rather than the bacilli of

the disease have come to be regarded as the villains of the plague epidemics. Yet in a way they thoroughly deserve their reputation. They are unlovable animals that share some characteristics with human beings: thus both are omnivores that on occasion eat their own kind; unlike most mammals they recognise neither closed breeding seasons nor geographical restraint; they indulge in racial prejudices (the brown rat preys when possible on its black cousins); they combine to fight as armies; if rats are put into a cage and allowed to multiply their offspring will presently begin to kill each other; and finally, rats and men are able to live in a wider range of climates than any other animal, so that they have taken over the world as their parish.

Plague is carried by two species of rat. The black, sewer rat is comparatively domesticated, having lived in close contact with man in houses and on ships since ancient times. The brown rat is a fiercer cousin which only migrated out of Asia during the fifteenth century AD. It then colonised Europe so effectively that its elimination required the resource of such legendary figures as the pied piper of Hamelin. And the sturdier brown rats have fought a running battle with their black relations until the latter faced extermination.

Throughout modern history the horrors of plague so sharply impressed themselves on men's minds that it was known simply as 'the pest' and became a favourite literary theme. Thus in his *Decameron*, Boccaccio describes a group, of fugitives from the plague in Florence who whiled away their exile for ten days (hence the book's title) by exchanging stories, most of which were licentious.

Plague usually appears in pandemics, that is epidemics which affect large areas of the world. The Bible refers to one such visitation (in Samuel I, V and VI) which 'smote [the Philistines] with buboes* . . . in their secret parts', caused

* A bubo is a glandular swelling in the groins and arm-pits of man. They were translated in the English version as 'emerods' meaning 'swellings'. The word was later applied to haemorrhoids which are, of course, quite different.

'deadly destruction throughout all the city' and was
attended by many deaths among the 'mice that mar the
land', an early reference to the association of plague with a
high mortality among rodents.

Outbreaks of plague erupted periodically in ancient
Rome and led to mass conversions to Christianity. For the
preachers of the early Church showed a real interest in
relieving the miseries of sickness, the majority of Christ's
miracles were of a medical nature, and He gave his disciples
'power ... to cure all diseases', a dispensation which
appealed to people living under the threat of a new visitation of plague.

One of the most lethal outbreaks of the 'pest' reached
Byzantium in AD 542 and spread out to affect the whole of
the civilised world. There is some dispute as to its starting
point: according to Edward Gibbon, Egypt and Ethiopia
were 'the original source and seminary of the plague'. If
Gibbon was correct we may assume that the infection spread
to parts of East Africa, and certainly Uganda subsequently
became an endemic area, the infection being kept alive in
wild rodents. Constantinople was so badly infected by the
'Justinian Plague' of 542 that there was a scarcity of grave
diggers and the surviving citizens had no option but to stuff
the abundant corpses into the towers along the city's walls.
The outbreak defeated the Emperor Justinian's attempts to
restore the Roman empire to its earlier limits. Instead,
the plague set his empire on the long, slow decline which
culminated in the fall of Constantinople in 1453. The outbreak was ultimately responsible for the shift in world
power from the Mediterranean basin to western Europe.

The next outbreak of plague was no less catastrophic. It
occurred in Europe during 1348–9 and was known as the
'Black Death'; the name is believed to refer either to the
dark spots of haemorrhage under the victims' skin or to the
deadly character of the pandemic.

It was this disaster which gave rise to the nursery rhyme,
Ring-a-ring o'roses; the ring represents the circle of red spots

which appear on some plague victims, the posies stands for the posies of flowers and herbs carried to ward off infection (and are still in fact carried by the Monarch, senior officers of the City of London Guilds at public appearances, and judges), 'a-tishoo' represents the sneezing of patients whose lungs were affected, while 'all fall down' signified their sudden deaths. The Black Death is believed to have killed about twenty-five million people, a quarter of Europe's inhabitants, and it led to far-reaching economic and social changes. Terror and panic gripped the whole of Christendom when it appeared and attempts to prevent a recurrence led to such phenomena as the craze for self-flagellation, the dancing mania, and the Children's Crusade. Domestic preventive measures included total abstinence from loose women and alcohol and 'listening to beautiful music and songs'. There was also a vogue for wearing medals of the patron saints of the disease, St Roch being particularly favoured; he was usually depicted on medallions with a bubo in his groin, although the swelling, for the sake of decorum, was sometimes shifted to his thigh. In the Balkans billy goats were confidently accommodated in dwelling places in the belief that their powerful smell discouraged the plague germ, while the remote village of Oberammergau took an entirely different prophylactic line by mounting regular Passion plays, hoping that such diligent piety would fend off further visitations.

No effective remedy for plague was known; in any case this mattered little since physicians were loth to visit the infected, perhaps less for fear of catching the infection than because there was little chance of collecting fees since the patients would surely die within a few days. Still, many quack remedies were sold including scented alcholic infusions of herbs, one of which has survived as 'eau de Cologne'. Tobacco smoking was later recommended as a preventative during the Plague of London, and boys at Eton were whipped for not smoking. Pepys chose to chew tobacco. Persons accused of spreading the infection were tortured to death in Italy, while Burgundians engaged in pogroms on the approach of plague. The Venetians more sensibly (though the measure was erroneously based on astronomical notions) confined all travellers to the city on an island in the lagoon for forty days, and in doing so gave us the word 'quarantine'.*

Outbreaks of plague continued to scourge Europe. Some led to unlikely consequences. Thus during the fourteenth century the 'pest' wiped out the Viking colony of Greenland, and so delayed the discovery of America for a hundred years. London was sorely affected during 1665, and both Pepys and Defoe, who survived the pestilence, left us graphic accounts of its manifestations. On government instructions special 'searchers' in England were engaged to compile weekly 'bills of mortality' which reflected the death rates in various parts of the kingdom. Later on these became more regularised and developed into the science of natural statistics.

But presently plague turned its back on Europe, and the reasons for its doing so have been widely debated. Possibly an improvement in domestic architecture which excluded rats from houses was responsible. Equally likely was the adoption of sea rather than land routes for world trade, or the replacement of black rats which frequented the ships by the hardier brown rats which are less susceptible to infection. But if Europe was spared the plague bacillus, towards the end of the nineteenth century the 'pest' won new and more prodigious victories in Asia and America. One of the worst outbreaks occurred in India during 1885 when an estimated million and a half persons died.

We have no knowledge of the extent of plague in tropical Africa prior to the European conquest, other than that it

---

*The forty-day term for quarantine may, however, be of biblical origin. There are several instances of this period being imposed as a penance, expiation or purification. The flood lasted forty days (Gen. VII), Moses was on the Mount for this period (Exodus XXIV), and Jesus fasted for forty days.

persisted in endemic form in Uganda. Then sporadic cases began to appear in African ports to which rats had carried the infection from visiting ships. But presently, as railway networks extended, the plague was carried inland. There, as their original rat hosts died off, the fleas transferred the infection to wild rodents whence it was from time to time transmitted to human beings who came into contact with them, particularly skinners and trappers.

Then in 1907 a more extensive outbreak occurred in Accra and spread up-country, causing over three hundred deaths. Lagos was twice affected during the 1920s and the infection reached as far north as Kano, where one European doctor and two nurses attending the sick died from the disease. Plague in East Africa also increased during the first three decades of this century. Twenty-five thousand deaths from the 'pest' were recorded from Uganda and Kenya during the period 1913–19. In 1926 the figure had dropped to one thousand eight hundred and forty and to a similar number during 1927. Most of the Ugandan cases occurred among people working in cotton fields where they were infected by wild rodents. In 1929–30 Kenya reported one thousand seven hundred and twenty-two cases while the Congo is known to have suffered more severely, but after 1930 the incidence of plague decreased. The 'pest' appeared in Botswana during 1944 after a drought drove infected jerbils (wild jerboa-like rodents) into contact with semi-domesticated mice, and their fleas passed on the germs to human beings. Mombasa has also been affected by passing ships, while infected rodents in coastal regions of Angola have been carried into the far interior along the Benguela railway.

The organism responsible for plague is a stubby bacillus, which was first identified by a Frenchman, Alexander Yersin (1863–1943), during an outbreak in Hong Kong in 1894. The life history of the germ was subsequently worked out by a score of scientific laboratories. Within recent years treatment with antibiotics and development of an effective vaccine have lessened the incidence of plague in tropical Africa.

It was long appreciated that outbreaks of plague were preceeded by a heavy mortality among rats and mice. The black sewer rat is a zealous traveller which frequents ships and docks, and this is the favoured host of both fleas and the plague bacillus. It was these rats which brought plague to African ports. Rats also travel with bales of wool and cotton, and before the maritime revolution the 'pest' was usually spread by caravans travelling along overland trade routes.

The risks to group survival of parasites responsible for human disease are well demonstrated by those affecting the fortunes of the plague bacillus. Its perpetuation largely depends on the maintenance of the organisms' transmission by a series of fleas to a series of rats. This circulation, however, sometimes breaks down under conditions which either increase the germs' virulence to rats or the fleas' fertility. There is some evidence that such developments occur during spells of unusual weather such as extremes of temperature or humidity. In either case a large die-off of rats results, and the fleas carrying plague are obliged to seek out alternative hosts, either other rodents or human beings. If the latter, an outbreak of human plague will occur. Even then the bacillus has a second line of attack, for its enjoys a reserve method of transmission which is not based on fleas: the bacilli lodge in the lungs of some human victims from which they can be directly passed on to other people in the breath, especially when coughing or talking.

Human plague thus appears in two clinical forms. The common type is termed bubonic plague since it is character-ised by the early appearance of buboes. It carries a mortality of about fifty per cent. The second form, pneumonic plague, occurs when the organism affects the human lungs. Pneumonic plague was invariably fatal until the appearance of modern antibiotics.

When outbreaks of plague occur, poisoned rat-baits are extensively used to limit the disease; insecticide dusting of persons likely to carry fleas is also practised as a preventive measure, while ships visiting ports are ordered to moor some distance from wharves to prevent rats coming ashore. In addition a strict quarantine of six days is imposed on persons travelling from plague-stricken areas. Yet despite such precautions the threat of new visitations of the 'pest' to Africa is always present and can only be avoided by constant watchfulness on the part of the public health authorities.

*   *   *

Since earliest times cholera has been endemic in the Ganges basin and in China. Then, during 1816, some change overtook the cholera germs, the bacteria of curved shape named vibrios which were later identified by Robert Koch in 1883. As if suddenly acquiring more aggressive powers it gave rise to serious epidemics in Europe and Asia, with smaller outbreaks in tropical Africa.

No one knows what precise factor increased the virulence of the cholera vibrio and changed it into a vicious killer bent upon territorial expansion; possibly a mutation occurred which resulted in the formation of toxins more dangerous than previously to its only host, man. The new-found aggressiveness was greatly assisted by the patterns of world trade imposed by Great Britain at the end of the Napoleonic wars.

It is convenient at this point to identify some of the great cholera pandemics of last century. These global extensions included the Middle East, Europe and finally America, during four separate periods: 1816–23, 1826–37, 1842–62, and 1865–75; each included 'side-show' forays into Black Africa. The African epidemics were carried to the east coast by ships from India, while the inland ranges of the first three were limited to those of the Arab caravans reaching into the interior, an example of the restriction on the spread of disease by the poor intracontinental communications existing in tropical Africa before the European conquest. During the 1816 pandemic, cholera in Africa was limited to the coastal hinterland of Tanzania; in that of 1826 the coastal regions of Somalia and Kenya were affected; during the third pandemic, cholera again affected Somalia and was carried inland almost to the Great Lakes from the Kenya-Tanzanian coast, and this pattern was repeated during the 1865 pandemic. This last major outbreak of cholera extended into West Africa from Morocco and gained a temporary base round the Gambia River. Minor outbreaks later occurred outside Asia without affecting tropical Africa, but a serious pandemic which began in the Celebes reached Africa again during 1970.

Cholera is an alarming disease. Once infected the patient is struck with violent diarrhoea, agonising cramps and frantic thirst. These symptoms are caused by the germ's release of a toxin which literally shreds the lining of the lower bowel. Death may occur within two hours of the onset. Macabre sequels to a fatal attack of cholera include the high temperature maintained for some hours by the corpse, and the post-mortem muscular contractions which suggest that the body is still alive. During an epidemic the mortality rate may be as high as fifty per cent. Those who are not attacked probably owe their lives to a high acid content of their gastric juices which destroys the germs before they reach the intestines.

Cholera epidemics are most likely to occur when the infections reach a group of susceptible victims who are crowded together following drought or famine, and liable to panic and so spread the infection. Unusual weather conditions of high humidity and heat also favour the spread of the disease. Some of the survivors from an attack of cholera become carriers of the germ and contribute to its survival. Cholera never appears, for some reason, in mountainous country.

An English doctor, John Snow, was the first man to demonstrate the method of transmission of cholera. He was practising in Soho in London during the middle of last century and when the disease struck, Snow drew a map of the Golden Square area of Soho which had become badly affected by the disease and on it marked the position of the houses where some five hundred deaths had occurred. He noticed that these homes stood in a tight cluster round a public water point in Broad Street only a few hundred yards from Golden Square. Snow reasoned that this water must be the source of the infection and on 8th September 1848 arranged for the handle of the pump to be removed. Almost miraculously no more cases occurred in the vicinity.

Snow had thus neatly demonstrated that cholera was a water-borne disease. This was recognised as a milestone in the development of preventive medicine, and the site of the pump in Broad Street was marked by a coloured cobble. No other memorial was raised to John Snow, though a nearby public house was named for him, and perhaps this was the sort of tribute he would have preferred.

When cholera came to Africa, its people knew no remedy except flight, and thus greatly facilitated its extension. According to Sir Richard Burton, Arab merchants in East Africa treated themselves with opium and locally distilled spirits. In other parts of the world, sips of Condy's fluid (sodium potassium permanganate) enjoyed a therapeutic vogue. Many secret remedies against cholera were put up for sale, particularly after the disease reached the United States where it greatly enhanced the financial expectations of quack therapists.

A major step in the treatment of the disease occurred in 1915 when Sir Leonard Rogers began giving weak intravenous solutions of common table salt to his cholera patients and so replaced the loss of fluids and minerals which had occurred. This was rational therapy and the ingredients were gradually elaborated with immense saving of life. Infusions of fluid into the veins requires trained staff but it was found that reasonably good results came from fluid replacement on the lines already described in the treatment of different diarrhoeal infections. As with so many other diseases, the appearance during the past forty years of increasingly effective antibiotics has revolutionised the curative treatment of cholera.

Yet prevention still requires our attention. Essentially it depends on the provision of safe water, the enforcing of effective quarantine regulations, and vaccination of people at risk from cholera. Now the tide has turned in the fight: like a defeated army cholera has withdrawn to its old Asiatic bases, and for the present Africa seems safe from its onslaught.

*   *   *

From time to time influenza swept through sub-Saharan Africa, and the most serious visitation was the 'Spanish flu' epidemic of 1918. It was so called because of its supposed place of origin, although in fact it began in Canton. It descended on Europe in the summer of 1918, and reached the West African coast during August, spreading rapidly inland. During the next two years almost the entire world was affected, and only St Helena, New Guinea and a few islands in the Pacific were spared. Fifty per cent of the world's population, perhaps half a billion people, caught the infection; it claimed over twenty million lives, more than the number killed during the 1914–18 war. In India alone the deaths exceeded twelve million.

It was the most lethal outbreak of disease in world history, worse even than the Justinian plague and the Black Death. One of its tragic features was that it was most dangerous to the young and vigorous, while older people suffered to a far lesser extent.

The pandemic is still spoken of in Africa with awe, but we possess comparatively few records of the outbreaks. In Southern Rhodesia it chiefly affected people living in towns or working in mines. Those who became ill fled to their villages and quickly spread the infection through the entire colony. Only a few isolated rural communities escaped. So serious was the disruption of life in Southern Rhodesia that normal activities – social, administrative and economic – in effect stopped. All major mines closed down for want of workers and hospitals became so overcrowded that private houses were opened as makeshift nursing homes. About ten per cent of those affected died. In the whole of Black Africa about a million people perished.

When possible, the Rhodesian Africans sought help from their traditional healers, but many victims knew of no better remedy than cold water bathing which probably did more harm than good. The medical services, already strained by war-time conditions, broke down in the crisis, and many rural Africans had to rely on the homely remedies provided by white settlers. They prescribed quinine and epsom salts when available, but draughts of paraffin mixed with eucalyptus and a few drops of Friar's Balsom were believed by the patients to be more effective, and there was a run on axle-grease which could be used to poultice the sufferers' chests. In the mines, of 32,766 men employed, a total of 3,629 are known to have died from the infection.

In East Africa the death toll was so high that a doctor lamented that 'one cannot believe that this people will ever recover'. West Africa was equally badly affected. Eighty per cent of the inhabitants of Calabar, for instance, went down with the flu, while in British Cameroons, which the disease reached during November 1918, a reported 35,000 people died of the infection out of a total population of 153,360.

In Ghana all churches, schools and other meeting places were closed with little obvious effect, and where possible free milk and drugs were distributed to those suffering from it. Influenza epidemics reappeared during 1957 and 1968, but neither were so deadly as that of 1918.

The influenza virus appears in a large number of different strains. All exhibit astonishingly agile genetic shift and drift, and considerable immunological variation. In consequence mutants with high survival values are always available whenever the parental strain is threatened. In addition the virus reproduces so rapidly that the whole process of evolution seems to have been accelerated.

Accordingly the virus readily adapts to the tardier defence mechanisms of its human prey and appears in a variety of clinical syndromes which are not labelled with scientific names but with homelier ones like 'Russian flu' because of their assumed territorial origin.

The viruses of influenza are under continuous surveillance coordinated by the World Health Organisation, and vaccines are prepared from isolated strains of the virus most likely to be the cause of any outbreak. Without doubt antibiotics reduce the severity of complications of the infection, but they have no effect on the responsible virus itself.

*   *   *

Older generations of medical practitioners in Africa were impressed by two related facts: one was that the people suffered unduly from the cold during winter seasons, tending then to huddle together and to close every possible source of ventilation; the second was that as a consequence of their sensitivity to cold weather, they suffered severely from cerebro-spinal meningitis, commonly known as 'spotted fever', which raged periodically through their land.

Spotted fever causes inflammation of the membranes (the meninges) which surround and protect the brain and spinal cord. The disease appears to be a comparative newcomer to the world; it was first recognised during 1805 in Geneva. Soon afterwards it affected troops in south-west France and presently appeared in Ireland during the potato famine of 1848. Since then it has been found in all parts of the world and is particularly prevalent among those people living in closed quarters like army barracks, prisons and schools. Epidemic meningitis apparently first appeared in Africa in 1900 when it was diagnosed on the west coast, and it spread quickly across the continent. Since then all parts of sub-Saharan Africa have suffered from extensive outbreaks, most of them occurring during winter. The great West African epidemic of the 1930s started in the Sudan during 1930 and finally reached Sierra Leone and Gambia

in 1941. In Ghana meningitis occurs in the cool dry season
and stops abruptly with the rains.

The responsible germ is a rounded bacterium or coccus,
and was identified by Edwin Klebs in Zurich. It soon became
apparent that many persons harboured the coccus in their
noses and yet remained perfectly healthy even during an
outbreak of meningitis. Such people are 'carriers' of
the disease, periodically passing on the germ to susceptible
contacts when coughing or sneezing and when the secretions of the victims' noses have dried up due to colds, thus
removing an effective barrier to infection. Epidemics may
reach disastrous proportions and carry a mortality rate of
over seventy per cent.

The onset of cerebro-spinal meningitis is startlingly sudden. The patient complains of a severe headache and stiff
neck, runs a high temperature, while red spots appear scattered over the belly. Convulsions occur during the terminal
stages of the disease.

The appearance of meningitis in the remote districts of
Africa imposed great responsibility on the medical officers
in charge. Their chief problem lay in ensuring the isolation
of all patients and contacts, and it was no easy task. The
doctors would trudge or cycle along the winding paths of
Africa to the affected villages and find that the whole life of
the community had come to a stop. The huts would be filled
by stiff-backed patients, utterly careless of the world around
them, mutely accepting their fate, refusing any help. To
prevent spread of the infection it was imperative that all
meningitis cases be moved into a bush camp where they
slept out in the open. It took time to organise such camps
and to persuade the patients to move into them; sometimes
the exercise required help from the local police, but it was
the only way to stop an epidemic.

Fortunately today, in the sulphonamides and antibiotics,
we possess effective remedies for preventing the spread of
the infection and curing patients, and they have reduced its
mortality to under ten per cent. But still in Africa medical

auxilliaries have an important part to play in reporting outbreaks of this dreaded disease to headquarters so that prompt steps may be taken to prevent its further spread.

*　　　*　　　*

To their medical officers, the colonial administrations throughout tropical Africa appeared to be far more concerned with epidemic infections than dealing with endemic diseases; they tended instead to regard the latter as necessary evils. As we have seen, the authorities had reacted energetically to the sudden appearance of sleeping sickness in Uganda as far back as 1901; and since then, whenever epidemics of meningitis and measles broke out in Africa, directives for controlling them poured out from medical headquarters. The officials there were particularly sensitive to outbreaks of smallpox, perhaps because there was an effective vaccine. The doctors in the bush greatly dreaded its occurrence, for as Sir Richard Burton had noted in 1860, smallpox was 'the most dangerous epidemic . . . which . . . sweeps at times like a storm of death over Africa'. Twenty years later Dr E.J. Southon of the London Missionary Society recorded that 'the average life of the males [at Unyamezi in East Africa] does not exceed twenty to twenty-five years' since most fell victims to smallpox, famines and fighting. In Uganda, C.J. Wilson of the Church Missionary Society recorded in 1887 that smallpox was 'one of the most fatal [diseases to which the Ganda are subject], coming at intervals in epidemics and carrying off thousands of victims; few attacked ever recover,' while as early as 1876 Dr James Christie had concluded that 'there is no disease in East Africa so fatal in its ravages as smallpox.'

Smallpox is a highly infectious disease which is spread by direct contact with a patient or with his clothes, bed linen and feeding utensils. The illness is ushered in by a high temperature; three days later purulent blisters develop over the body. Many patients will die at this stage; in those that recover the sores dry up and form scabs which finally drop off leaving disfiguring scars.

It is believed that smallpox originated either in India or in Central Africa – most probably in the latter. It is a very ancient disease well known in pharaonic Egypt. In 1979 the mummy of Rameses V, who died in 1157 BC at the age of forty, was carefully examined by American specialists. They reported that smallpox was 'written all over Rameses's face and body' in the form of yellowish blisters which exactly resembled the pocks of smallpox. Microscopy unfortunately failed to demonstrate the smallpox virus, but presumably this had shared death with Rameses, its earliest known victim.

Smallpox was probably the plague of Athens which was vividly described by Thucydides (c. 431 BC) though the epidemic has also been attributed to plague, typhus, a virulent form of measles and even anthrax. This outbreak is important to history since it demoralised the Athenians during their war with the Pelopennesians who subsequently ravaged Attica at will and destroyed the Athenian empire. Marcus Aurelius was a victim of smallpox. Returning crusaders reintroduced the infection to Europe, and smallpox became common in England during Tudor times. It increased its virulence towards the end of the seventeenth century, accounting for twenty-three per cent of the deaths in Britain. Sixty million people are believed to have succumbed to smallpox in Europe during the Thirty Years War (1618–1648). Queen Mary II of England died from smallpox in 1694, while the face of Louis XV before his death was so badly affected that he appeared to have two noses.

Records reveal that smallpox appeared in Japan about AD 980 and that the patients were treated by hanging red cloth curtaining around them, a form of therapy which was commonly practised in England until recent times.

Smallpox was introduced into Mexico during 1520 when Panfilo Narvaez landed at Vera Cruz in the wake of Cortes.

Among his followers was an African slave who had recently contracted the infection in San Domingo, smallpox having been carried there from Europe. Within a few years small-pox killed off over half the Aztec emperor's subjects, and this, more than any other factor, allowed the Spaniards' easy conquest of Mexico. The infection then spread to the Inca kingdom and was so disastrous that resistance to Pizarro's invasion which followed was minimal; after the conquest the ancient Inca gods abdicated, while their followers accepted the Spaniards as overlords and underwent mass conversion to Christianity. Smallpox also subsequently decimated the Indians of North America and played a large part in the United States' winning of the west.

Smallpox probably occurred in tropical Africa from earliest times, but some accounts suggest that it was rein-troduced by Arabs who crossed the Sahara during the eighth century AD. It was reported again in Africa during the tenth century although appearing in a comparatively mild form called *Variola minor*. It was well known on the Guinea Coast during the seventeenth century; and again was so mild that the few deaths recorded by a European traveller were, he said, caused by sepsis or 'sheer pain' due to the patients lying in 'dry sandy soil'. A smallpox epidemic was reported in Angola as early as 1627, the outbreak apparently having been provoked by the movement of refugees from Portuguese depredations. Another Angolan epidemic in 1793 similarly followed a punitive expedition undertaken by Portuguese troops into the interior. The more virulent form of smallpox – *Variola major* – appeared in Angola during 1864. The Africans called it 'Ki-ngongo' (great suffering) and sometimes 'Ki-beta' (great punish-ment). Its appearance may have been associated with an increasing export trade in wax and ivory. The disease carried a sixty per cent mortality and forty thousand fatal cases occurred in Luanda alone. Those victims who sur-vived, according to a Portuguese doctor, resembled 'mummies rather than human beings'. By the time of the general European conquest of Africa smallpox had become widespread. It was reported from most of the new African dependencies and caused particular concern to the German colonists in the Iringa district of modern Tanzania, since one third of the African inhabitants became infected. Only a little later Albert Cook warned that smallpox was a constant threat to the people of Uganda who suffered terribly from an epidemic in 1891. This had followed so quickly on the rinderpest that the Africans believed smallpox to be the human manifestation of this veterinary disease.

Smallpox became very prevalent in Nigeria during colonial times. Intercession for help against the infection was made to a god named Shopanna. Priests of the rite nursed smallpox victims in special huts and prescribed applications of various ointments to the sores; they also undertook disposal of the dead, and the burning of the infected clothing. The priests forbade large gatherings during epidemics and laid down special rules for the community which regulated inter-village travel.

Converts to Islam preferred a different therapy: they wrote verses from the Koran on parchment, then washed the ink into a cup and drank its contents. Variolation (the inoculation with pus from the pock of a smallpox victim) was commonly practised throughout old Africa. The pus was usually scratched into the skin. This resulted in what was generally a mild attack of smallpox, and thus conferred life-long immunity to the disease.

Thomas Bowdich, who travelled through modern Ghana during 1815 to make peace with the king of Ashanti, described the method of variolation practised there: 'they take the matter and puncture the person in seven places, both in the arms and legs. The sickness continues but a few days and rarely any person dies from it.' In fact the mortality from variolation or 'ingrafting' was between two and three per cent in Europe and the practice fell into disuse there after 1728.

Lady Mary Wortley Montague was responsible for popularising 'ingrafting' in England during 1721 after watching Turkish women introducing small amounts of smallpox 'matter' into the arms of healthy people. (She gained another niche in history by popularising the wearing of 'bloomers' by English women.) The Reverend Cotton Mather, better known for his rigid puritanism and stimulation of the witchcraft trials in Salem, almost simultaneously introduced variolation into the British North American colonies, having learned the technique from his Negro slaves.

Seventy years were to pass before Edward Jenner demonstrated a far safer way of preventing smallpox when he introduced vaccination. A medical practitioner in Gloucester, he had been impressed by the popular belief that milkmaids never contracted smallpox: indeed their immunity from facial scarring so contrasted with the pocks which blemished many other women, that it gave rise to the nursery rhyme:

> 'Where are you going to, my pretty maid?'
> 'I'm going a-milking, Sir' she said,
> 'What is your fortune, my pretty maid?'
> 'My face is my fortune, Sir' she said.

Jenner realised that the milkmaids' immunity to smallpox was due to their liability to contract cowpox, a mild illness related to smallpox which occurs in cattle. He took 'matter' from the pocks on the fingers of one of his cowpox patients and scratched it into the arm of a healthy boy. The boy duly went down with a mild attack of cowpox and thereafter resisted attempts to innoculate him with smallpox.

Jenner's vital demonstration in 1796 that immunity to smallpox could be achieved by 'vaccination' (the injection of cowpox pus) resulted in the disappearnce of smallpox where vaccination was practised. But the disease continued to rage through underdeveloped countries. Even during the 1950s an estimated twenty million cases were occurring in the world each year of which three million died and hundreds of thousands were blinded. In particular, the emerging African states found it impossible to provide protection against smallpox for all their people during the following decade.

During a sessional meeting at the World Health Organisation in 1958, however, the delegate of the USSR proposed that all the countries in the world united in a global campaign to eradicate smallpox. The campaign envisaged would transcend all barriers of nationality, language and tradition. The proposer believed that vaccination (and when necessary revaccination) of eighty per cent of the world's population could be achieved within the following four or five years, and that the infection would then die out.

The campaign began in January 1957 and was continued for the next ten years with excellent results in some countries but failed to reach the goal of total eradication. In 1966 the situation was re-examined; it was realised that the campaign had only been partly successful because of the limited financial resources of some of the participating nations. In particular four reservoirs of endemic smallpox persisted in tropical Africa alone. The WHO responded by intensifying the campaign after obtaining generous additional finances from the USA, USSR and other developed countries. By the late 1960s every nation in the world had become engaged again in the eradication programme.

The stress was now placed on surveillance. Reporting teams were trained to seek out smallpox patients, to isolate them and then vaccinate all contacts. They were provided with simple two-pronged lancets which held just enough lymph for successful vaccination and which were easily sterilised. At the same time mass vaccination campaigns for healthy subjects were mounted on a global scale, two hundred and fifty million doses being provided annually. By 1971 central and western Africa had been finally freed from the ancient scourge.

But the infection still clung to its last strongholds in the Horn of Africa and five Asiatic countries. Intense campaigning eliminated foci in the latter and finally smallpox was alive only in Ethiopia, where four hundred cases were reported during 1976. Unfortunately the success of vaccination campaigns had been jeopardised by civil war, famine and the movement of hordes of refugees.

All efforts were now concentrated on Ethiopia, and the country was declared free at last from smallpox in August 1976. But by then the infection had spilled over into Somalia and the medical teams moved on to this final objective. And on 26th October 1977 Ali Maow Maalin, a twenty-three-year-old hospital cook living in Merka near Mogadishu was the last case to be diagnosed as suffering from smallpox. He made a quick recovery and no more natural cases of the disease have occurred since then, though some technicians have become accidentally infected during laboratory experiments.

Smallpox is the first human disease ever eradicated by man. The only living smallpox viruses are confined now to glass vials held under strict security in the laboratories of six countries. The conquest of smallpox has been a notable victory for medicine. It represented a human ability to change the world for the better through the mutual cooperation and mobilisation of resources on a global scale; and the phrase 'bid the sickness cease' had gained new meaning.

Much of the credit for this triumph must go to Edward Jenner. He was greatly honoured during his lifetime, though not by the Royal College of Physicians in England who declined to make him a fellow unless he passed a test in the classics of ancient medical writers, a proposal which Jenner declined. In Russia the first child to be vaccinated was named Vaccinov and provided with free education in Jenner's honour; statues were raised to him in Kensington Gardens and Gloucester Cathedral, others at Boulogne and Brünn. He merits another one at Merca in tropical Africa where smallpox finally died.

It is worth noting that the virus of monkey pox is very like that of smallpox, and has occasionally infected man. It is, however, very unlikely to take the place of smallpox.

13

'Bid the Sickness Cease'

A NEW ERA in the history of tropical Africa opened in 1956 when Ghana attained its independence. Within twenty-five years colonialism was almost dead and fifty newly independent states had emerged in Africa.

After 1956 science gained some notable successes against tropical illnesses: smallpox was eliminated, the incidence of yaws declined to statistical insignificance, and life expectancy in Africa rose from 35.9 to 43.5 years (although this still compared badly with 70 years in more developed countries). But there had been disappointments too, especially in the field of malaria: during the middle 1960s it was confidently expected that the new insecticides would quickly eliminate the disease in tropical Africa, as had already occurred in Greece, Venezuela, Taiwan, Mexico, Sri Lanka, the tropical regions of the USSR and most of the West Indian islands. Yet by the end of the decade large endemic areas of malaria still persisted in the continent and indeed the incidence of malaria was rising. All the earlier talk of malaria eradication changed to discussion of methods of obtaining at least some tolerable reduction of the disease, and even these failed to produce results, so that today malaria is as prevalent as ever before. Unfortunately, so are many other diseases affecting the Africans.

Several factors contributed to the malaria anticlimax: many African dwellings were inaccessible to DDT spraying teams, their inhabitants were sometimes unco-operative, financial support for the malaria campaign dried up, and there was an inflationary rise in the price of insecticides and of the petrol which carried them to where they were needed. But a far more potent factor in defeating the malaria campaigns had been the unexpected complexity of the parasites responsible for the disease. Their variability allowed them to react successfully to each fresh therapeutic advance through the survival of strains resistant to the newly introduced drugs, and the frequency of these strains increased sufficiently rapidly to replace those which had been destroyed by each new remedy.

The hopes of vector control of tropical diseases by the modern insecticides were similarly frustrated by the appearance of resistant mosquitoes and other carriers. The emergence of resistant plasmodia and of DDT-proof mosquitoes provided Africa with bitter evidence of the continued appearance of new varieties of life; the defensive mechanisms so rapidly developed by pathogenic organisms were a grim reminder that evolution is never stationary, but is always progressing.

The failure of science to grapple successfully with the health crisis in tropical Africa is illustrated by a survey undertaken in Rwanda during 1973. It showed that even at this time three hundred children out of every thousand born would still die of disease before the age of five. Yet, despite such a loss, the survey also showed that the country was threatened by a dangerous population growth. This increase was caused by a recent decline in adult mortality and, more particularly, by an increasing birth-rate. For the average Rwandan woman bears between six and seven children, while the number in Kenya and other African states is over eight. This high birth-rate reflected an improvement in ante-natal care and also the people's fears for the future, for in Africa only a large family will insure against poverty in old age.

Other surveys have shown that the annual population growth rate in most African countries now exceeds 3.5 per cent. The estimated population of Africa rose from 278 million during the fifties to 380 million in 1976 and is expected to reach 580 million by the end of this century. The present 'swarming' of the people is continuing at a rate which exceeds the continent's capacity to increase food production, and the old gibe that medical men merely save lives in Africa so that their patients might starve to death begins to ring true. In consequence, most doctors have come to believe that restraint of birth is as important as restraint of death.

But Africa's population problem must finally be solved by the sociologists, and we are here concerned with the still unacceptable morbidity of Black Africa from diseases which are nearly all theoretically preventable. It would be wrong to attribute the existing high disease incidence in sub-Saharan Africa solely to genetic changes in pathogenic organisms of disease or in their vectors. Many other spoiling factors have been at work varying from a rise in the price of drugs to disastrous failure of the rains in many parts of the continent. But the sad fact remains that other contributions to the failure to banish disease from the continent are man-made. Independent African states have had to meet so many financial demands, particularly for national security, that they are not always able to give all the attention they wish to carrying out public health policies which are required. But more significant has been the replacement of democratic forms of government in many African countries by coups which installed dictatorships or rule by military juntas; these, if they are to survive, must expend their budgets on armaments rather than on health. And where there are soldiers and guns there will be fighting, refugees, a break-down in existing medical services and a widening spread of disease.

Few countries in Africa have suffered more than Zimbabwe from a political dispute which could have been solved peacefully. Caught up in a spiral of internal violence three-quarters of a million people were forced by contending armies to flee from their villages; of this number about one third took refuge in either Mozambique, Zambia or Botswana. Despite contributions from the UN High Commission, food in the refugee camps was very scarce;

clothing, blankets and shoes were desperately short, and medicines too were lacking. The refugees suffered especially from malaria, bilharzia, kwashiorkor and gastro-enteritis for which no drip therapy was available. One strange disease caused paralysis and screaming fits in young girls and this was thought to be of psychological origin. The doctors at one camp of twelve thousand refugees possessed only one stethoscope and two thermometers to deal with the situation. Most of the other displaced persons squatted where they could find transient accommodation beyond the fighting zones. Immunerable primary schools were forcibly closed during hostilities together with eighty secondary schools. Forty-four hospitals and many clinics were obliged to cease services to the sick. Only two doctors were able to work in an area previously served by eight. The International Red Cross reported that a million peasants and refugees within the country were suffering from malnutrition, and that tropical diseases were increasing unchecked.

As armed men roamed the countryside seeking out or avoiding each other, I had an opportunity to study the medical results of the fighting. Health services in the country prior to the war were accounted among the most efficient in Africa but now in many areas they disintegrated. Malaria control was the first to be affected, and then the bilharzial preventive measures were abandoned over large regions. The inhabitants of many parts of the country found themselves in a desperate condition: for years they had encountered no malaria and their immunity had lapsed; now they suffered severe attacks. Similarly bilharzia which had been partially contained, appeared again in a more virulent form, while tsetse flies carrying sleeping sickness returned to areas which had been previously freed.

The terrorised peasants were driven from their lands by fighting and intimidation, so ploughing and planting ceased. As food became short, many of the villagers drifted off to the towns where at least they would be sustained by the African sense of responsibility to extended families.

Infectious diseases, especially among children, increased dramatically. Before the fighting began, mobile units comprising a nursing sister and an assistant, both skilled in antenatal care and pediatrics, had ranged through the rural parts of the country, providing attention for the sick and pregnant women, checking signs of malnutrition in children, immunising them against diphtheria, tetanus, whooping cough, poliomyelitis, smallpox and measles. Their campaigns had eliminated diphtheria from most of Rhodesia and drastically curtailed the incidence of measles and other infectious diseases. After the withdrawal of the teams, infantile susceptibility to these infections rapidly increased. Diphtheria was the first to appear, followed in ominous sequence by most of the others, the health authorities becoming particularly concerned by the possibility of a devastating outbreak of poliomyelitis, which fortunately did not occur.

The Africans in Rhodesia also suffered severely from the breakdown in veterinary services. The dipping of cattle was prevented in many tribal lands by one or other of the fighting rival factions, and a million head of cattle perished unnecessarily from tick-borne disease. Since the value of each beast averaged $100, this loss meant that millions of dollars of African money simply disappeared. Outbreaks of foot and mouth disease put an end to the selling of meat and hides, and this too was reflected in a cash loss by innumerable traders. The practice of agriculture was limited and often disastrously disrupted by fighting; in many African regions fertilisation of lands, contour ridging and crop rotation were abandoned, resulting in a serious loss of food.

The war closed schools, and the threat from landmines and ambushes halted bus services, so that sick people could not reach the hospitals which still remained open. Perhaps the most sadly affected were the old people, blinded by cataract, who previously had eagerly sought the dramatic cures of surgery and were now immobilised. Shops were closed and food for sale disappeared. Even minimal prosperity in the midst of such poverty and suffering 'marked' the more well-to-do Africans, for soldiers of both forces stigmatised them as enemies of the people or collaborators. Those of them who were not killed were forced to close down their small rural businesses, maize mills and transport services; they then sunk into anonymity, studiously avoiding prominence and even mental resistance to either side. Accordingly, though the Africans grumbled together in their own family circles, they did not report any depredations against their villages to the rival headquarters. Fear stalked the land; acceptance of terror and fickle death sentences became the terrible norm.

I have written at some length about the tribulations which overcame an African people when war engulfs their country, and squanders their health and safety. But we must turn now to the factors which are presently working in Africa's favour in the field of medicine, and of them all, the establishment of the World Health Organisation whose efforts are particularly directed at improving health standards in less developed parts of the world, is by far the most promising.

The World Health Organisation was set up by the United Nations during 1948 and given a global mandate to develop international health. The organisation is supported by donations from member nations, and the sums expended have already been more than regained by the eradication of smallpox alone.

This Organisation believes that there can be no justification for the present world system which still withholds the gift of health from underdeveloped nations. One of its functions is to exert the maximum possible effort to break the vicious circle of poverty, ignorance and disease which for so long has retarded the development of the Africans. It is determined to attain their complete physical, intellectual and social well-being. This can only be effected by eradication of disease and by improvements in standards of hygiene and sanitation which in turn depends to a large extent on educating the people. In addition, the WHO provides assistance to communities throughout the world including those who have suffered from natural disasters ranging from famine to earthquakes. It also sponsors research in medicine and the training of medical and paramedical personnel. It is difficult to think of a more worthy policy. In particular the organisation is determined to support such diverse objectives as the elimination of poverty in Africa, the provision of safe drinking water and elementary sanitation to every community, and special education for women about family planning. The improvement of child health and immunisation services is also high on the list of priorities, and it has inaugurated a drive to promote literacy among all the people. In addition, the WHO sponsors medical research which so far as tropical Africa is concerned is directed at malaria, bilharzia, onchoceriasis, sleeping sickness and leprosy. The organisation is also fostering research into a disease named kala-azar or leishmaniasis: kala-azar in itself is not particularly harmful to African health but its investigation is likely to yield valuable information about the complex relations between parasites and the cells of the human body and thus assist in the search for new drugs and vaccines.

As we have seen, the medical approach to the diseases of Africa has gone through several phases: at first the emphasis was placed on empirical treatments, then it shifted to differentiation of the separate infections together with identification of their causal organisms and methods of transmission; this was followed by attempted elimination of the vectors of disease and interest in vaccines; subsequently the emphasis was switched to antibiotic therapy and the elimination of nutritional diseases. Today the emphasis is being placed on the problem of taking medicine to the African masses rather than care for the minority living in towns and cities who have access to modern hospitals with advanced treatment facilities.

The most interesting development in this approach to the health problems of Africa lies in the concept of primary health care. This lays stress on the prevention of illnesses rather than their treatment; it also provides for rehabilitation of those who have suffered from disease, together with education of the communities about prevalent illness and the provision of paramedical care for people living in remote areas. The health personnel are expected to send only seriously ill patients to central medical institutions.

The whole concept of primary care lies in taking health to the people in their villages rather than spending most of the medical budget on urban hospitals where a large proportion of medical personnel are at present employed. In Ghana for instance, eighty-nine per cent of nurses work in town hospitals and a mere five-and-a-half per cent serve the rural populations.

The primary care concept envisages stationing non-physician, paramedical staff at rural centres serving about five thousand people. These health workers and inspectors are trained for about three months at a central depot where they are taught the signs and symptoms of the common ailments they are likely to meet, and the treatment of simple wounds, general pains, malaria, diarrhoea, anaemia and worm infestations. They are also instructed in handling simple drugs like aspirin, worm remedies, and chloroquine (although warned that this still valuable drug, if wrongly prescribed, may lead to inflammation of the eyes and mental instability). They are made familiar too with the technique of oral rehydration for diarrhoeal diseases.

In addition, the health workers are expected to educate the community about the prevention of the prevalent diseases in their district, advise on the virtues of longer spacing between children, organise community work which is geared to local health problems (such as providing proper drainage for the village) and to identify and co-operate with the traditional birth assistants and herbalists.

Every year health auxilliaries should return to the training centre for a refresher course and to learn more advanced methods of therapy such as the setting up of intravenous infusions. These 'medics' are essentially multi-purpose and fulfil many duties other than active treatment. Thus they arrange for their villages to be kept clean, identify disease sources such as stagnant pools and garbage in the area, supervise the local water supply, encourage the villagers to grow supplementary food stuffs in their lands, and organise regular visits by children to health centres for immunisation against diphtheria, whooping cough, polio-myelitis, tuberculosis, tetanus and measles. Their duties also should include educating the women in possible risks to their own health and that of their children, training health personnel, keeping vital statistics of morbidity and mortality in the villages and maintaining watch for any outbreaks of infectious disease in their area which may require the attention of medical headquarters.

The rural health workers are controlled from head-quarters, but a local committee is usually set up to assist them. This committee usefully includes the local religious leader, a prominent business man, a representative of the village women, a youth leader, and an elected representative from the community.

The emphasis of primary care then is placed more on preventive medicine and rehabilitation than on curative care, but the community worker should be properly supported by an efficient ambulance service which will take any seriously ill patients to back-up hospitals where they can receive more specialised attention.

Health personnel are encouraged to be on good terms with the traditional healers in their districts. These medi-cine men often specialise in a single field, and include herbalists, general therapists, psychotherapists, bone set-ters, practitioners of first aid surgery, and birth attendants. The herbalists are practical botanists, and the medical authorities in some African states now encourage them to send their favoured potions to headquarters for scientific assessment of their curative qualities. In practice several effective herbal cures are recognised in Africa today for diseases ranging from herpes to diabetes and epilepsy. One commentator has summed up the aims of health care for Africa succinctly as:

> Village clinics before city hospitals,
> local herb remedies before imported drugs,
> vaccines before kidney machines,
> latrines before antibiotics.

While strongly supporting the concept of primary health care, the WHO has also rightly laid great emphasis on the importance of reducing the very high incidence of malnutrition still occurring in tropical Africa especially among children. Malnutrition appears to be an essentially human condition and perhaps it is man-made since it is uncommon in game but often seen in domestic animals. Accordingly the Organisation has given great encouragement to the education of the masses on the causes and effects of deficiency diseases. They are taught that the human body can only remain healthy if it takes three different types of food: carbohydrates for energy, protein for body building, and fat to provide heat. The body also needs an adequate intake of vitamins and minerals for general well-being. The WHO deprecates the dietary taboos which are still practised in various parts of Africa: for instance some pregnant women will not eat eggs lest they make their children dumb and bald; they may shun fish which is supposed to give the baby worms, or milk because this inflames the mother's breasts; elsewhere rich food is believed to make their babies too large for easy delivery, and meat to increase bleeding after labour. The WHO preaches the virtues of breast feeding, pointing out that this provides the best possible nourishment for the baby and protects it against infections, particularly the dreaded diarrhoea.

The commonest deficiency disease still to be seen in Africa is kwashiorkor which is so dangerous during infancy as to merit brief re-emphasis here. It is caused by an inadequate intake of calories, proteins and of vitamins A, B_2, and C; their deficiency so greatly reduces an infant's resistance to infection that fifty per cent of affected children will die before the age of three.

Great benefit for tropical Africa is also expected to flow from WHO's encouragement of medical research on the continent. There are now twenty-five medical schools in sub-Saharan Africa, all capable of valuable research work, but they tend still to be under-staffed, under-equipped and under-funded. These restraints will only be overcome when greater incentives are provided for scientists and research workers, for at present it appears difficult to provide them with remuneration equivalent to that obtained in private practice. Africa needs the creation of an international body of health workers in politically stable states of the continent, and so far insufficient impetus to this concept has been provided. Nevertheless the WHO, encouraged by its recent victory over smallpox, is determined to eradicate disease from all countries of the third world, and its stated objective is now the attainment of 'health for all by the end of the century'. It must move fast to attain this goal in tropical Africa where medical problems are increasing, where too many of its people still lack such elementary facilities as clean drinking water and proper sanitation, and where the prevalence of several communicable and parasitic diseases is spreading.

The problems are daunting, the work to bring health to Africa will be arduous, but the prize is high yet attainable. World opinion is coming to regard the health situation in Africa as an offence against civilisation, and the Africans are facing the future with more confidence than they ever felt before, knowing that the United Nations and particularly the World Health Organisation are well aware of their problems and resolved to rectify them. Yet African governments must act with great wisdom in translating medical theory into practice, and this can only be accomplished in a continent at peace within itself.

Africa today is very different from the Africa of the past. It has been launched into an irreversible social revolution which has already initiated the transition from an emphasis on rural subsistence farming to industrialisation and urbanisation.

With independence, Africa found its soul as it took its place in world affairs and began to move from a colonial past into a future of her own making. That future must be one which will attain her peoples' fundamental right, in the phrase of the World Health Organisation, of 'Health for all by the year 2000'.

The attainment of that goal will require the full exploitation of Black Africa's human skills and cultural resources which for so long have lain unused. David Livingstone, that great lover of the African peoples, used to sigh that 'the day for Africa has yet to come'. As I write this chapter, towards the end of 1981, just a hundred years after the inception of the European conquest of the continent, that splendid event does not seem very far distant.

Bibliography

Beck, J.W., & Davies, J.E., *Medical Parasitology*, St Louis, 1976.

Boyd, *Sir* John, 'Sleeping Sickness, the Castellani-Bruce Controversy', *Notes and Records of the Royal Society*, 1973, *28*, 93.

Boyle, J., *A Practical Medico-Historical account of the western coast of Africa*, Lond., 1831.

Brabazon, J., *Albert Schweitzer*, Lond., 1976.

British Medical Journal, vol. 282, No. 6278, p. 1735. Leading article 'Yellow Fever – cause for concern'.

Bruce-Chwatt, L.J., 'Problems of Medical Control in Africa' in proceedings of Conference on *Malaria in Nigeria*, 24–27 Nov. 1975.

Carman, J.A., *A Medical History of Kenya*, Lond., 1976.

Cartright, F.F., *Disease and History*, Lond., 1972.

Castellani, A., *Microbes, Men and Monarchs*, Lond., 1960.

Castellani, A., & Chalmers, A.J., *Manual of Tropical Medicine*, Lond., 1919.

Clarke, E., *Modern Methods in the History of Medicine*, Athlone Press, 1971.

Clarke, J.I., *Population geography in developing countries*, Ox., 1971.

Clegg, A.C., & Clegg, P.C., *Man against disease*, Lond., 1973.

Cloudsley-Thompson, J.L., *The Zoology of Tropical Africa*, Lond., 1969.

Cloudsley-Thompson, J.L., *Insects and History*, Lond., 1977.

Clyde, D.F., *History of the Medical Services of Tanganyika*, Dar es Salaam, 1962.

Cockburn, A., *The Evolution and Eradication of Infectious Diseases*, Balt., 1963.

Cowper, S.G., *A Synopsis of African Bilharziasis*, Lond., 1971.

Crosby, A.W., *The Columbian Exchange*, Westport, 1972.

Curtin, P., Feiermans, S., Thompson, L., & Vansina, J., *African History*, Lond., 1978.

Curtin, P.D., *The Image of Africa*, Madison, 1964.

Darlington, C.D., *The Evolution of Man and Society*, 1969.

Davidson, B., *The African Past*, Lond., 1964.

Davies, J.N.P., 'The cause of Sleeping Sickness', *E.A. Medical Journal*, March and April, 1962.

Davies, J.N.P. 'The Development of Scientific Medicine in the

African kingdom of Bunyoro-Kitara', *Medical History*, 3, 47, 1959.

De Kruif, P., *Microbe Hunters*, N.Y., 1926.

Duggan, A.J., 'Tropical Medicine', *British contribution to medical science*, ed. Gibson, W.C., Lond., 1971.

Duggan, A.J., 'An Historical perspective', *The African trypanosomiasis*, ed. Mullgan, H.W., Lond. 1970.

Fiennes, R., *Man, Nature and Disease*, Lond., 1964.

Ford, J., *The Role of the Trypanosomiases in African Ecology*, Ox., 1971.

Foster, W.D., *A History of Parasitology*, Lond., 1965.

Foster, W.D., *Sir Albert Cook*, 1978.

Gale, A.H., *Epidemic Diseases*, Pelican, 1959.

Galton, F., *Art of Travel*, Lond., 1872.

Gann, L.H., & Duggan, P., *Burden of Empire*, Lond., 1967.

Gear, J.H.S. (ed.), *Medicine in a Tropical Environment*, Symposium, R.S.A., 1976.

Gelfand, M., *Medicine and Custom in Africa*, Lond., 1964.

Gelfand, M., *Tropical Victory*, C.T., 1953.

Gelfand, M., *Witch Doctor*, Lond., 1964.

Gelfand, M., *The Spiritual Beliefs of the Shona*, Sby, 1977.

Glemser, B., *The Long Safari*, Lond., 1970.

Goodwin, L.G., & Duggan, A.J., *A New Tropical Hygiene and Human Biology*, Lond., 1979.

Grove, A.T., *Africa*, OUP, 1978.

Hailey, Lord, *An African Survey*, Lond., 1957.

Hallett, R., *Africa to 1875*, Mich., 1970.

Hallett, R., *Africa since 1875*, Mich., 1974.

Hallett, R., *The Penetration of Africa*, Lond., 1965.

Harrison, G., *Mosquitoes, Malaria and Man*, Lond., 1978.

Hartwig, G.W., & Patterson, K.D., *Disease in African History*, Duke Univ., 1978.

Henschen, F., *The History of Diseases*, Lond., 1966.

Horton-Smith, C., ed., *Biological Aspects of the transmission of Disease*, Lond., 1957.

Hunter, J.M., 'River Blindness in Nangodi, Northern Ghana', *Geographical Review*, 96, 398, 1966.

Hyam, R., *Britain's Imperial Century*, Lond., 1976.

Kean, B.H., Mott, K.E., & Russell, A.J., *Tropical Medicine & Parasitology, Classic Investigations*, 2 vols., Lond., 1978.

Kimble, G.H.T., *Tropical Africa*, N.Y., 1960.

Kingsley, M.H., *West African Studies*, 3rd ed., Lond., 1964.

Konczacki, Z.A., & J.M., *An Economic History of Tropical Africa*, Lond., 1977.

Lapage, G., *Animals parasitic in Man*, N.Y., 1963.
Lechevalier, H.A., & Solotorovsky, M., *Three centuries of Microbiology*, N.Y., 1965.
Lewis, R., & Foy, Y., *The British in Africa*, Lond., 1971.
Lloyd, C., *The Search for the Niger*, Lond., 1973.
Lumsden, W.H.R., 'Some Episodes in the History of African Trypanosomiasis', *Proc. R. Soc. of Medicine*, 1974, 8, 789.
Lystad, R.A., (ed.), *The African World*, Lond., 1965.
Maclean, U., *Magical Medicine*, Lond., 1971.
Manson-Bahr, Sir P., 'The Story of Malaria', *Int. Rev. Trop. Med.*, 1963, 2, 329.
Manson-Bahr, P.H., and Alcock, A., *The Life and Work of Sir Patrick Manson*, Lond., 1927.
Martin, D. and Johnson, P., *The Struggle for Zimbabwe*, Lond., 1981.
McKelvey, J.R., jnr., *Man against Tsetse*, Lond., 1973.
NcNeill, W.H., *Plagues and People*, Ox., 1977.
Mégroz, R.L., *Ronald Ross*, Lond., 1931.
Nash, T.A.M., *Africa's Bane, the Tsetse Fly*, Lond., 1969.
Newby, E., *World Atlas of Exploration*, Lond., 1975.
Ngubane, H., *Body and Mind in Zulu Medicine*, Lond., 1977.
Nuttall, G.H.F., 'Forty Years of Parasitology and Tropical Medicine', *Background to Modern Science*, ed. Needham, J., & Pagel, W., Camb., 1938.
Parry, E.H.O., ed., *Principles of Modern Medicine in Africa*, Ox., 1976.
Patterson, K.D., 'Disease and Medicine in African History', *History in Africa*, 1974, I. 142.
Plumb, J.H., *Men and Places*, Lond., 1963.
Prothero, R.M., *Migrants and Malaria*, Lond., 1965.
Ross, Sir R., *Memoirs*, Lond., 1923.
Russell, P.F., *Man's Mastery of Malaria*, Lond., 1953.
Sabben-Clare, E.E., Bradley, D.J., & Kirkwood, K., (eds.), *Health in Tropical Africa during the Colonial Period*, Ox., 1980.
Schram, R., *A History of the Nigerian Health Services*, Ibadan, 1971.
Scott, D., *Epidemic Diseases in Ghana, 1901–1960*, Lond., 1965.
Scott, H.H., *A History of Tropical Medicine*, (2 vols.), Lond., 1939.
Service, M.W., 'A short History of early Medical Entomology', *Journal of Medical Entomology*, 14, (6) 603. 1978.
Severin, T., *The African Adventure*, Lond., 1973.
Singer, C., & Ashworth Underwood, E., *A Short History of Medicine*, Ox., 1962.
Sinnie, M., *Ancient African Kingdoms*, Norwich, 1965.
Stamp, L.D., *The Geography of Life and Death*, Lond., 1964.

Stanley, H.M., *The Congo and the Founding of its Free State*, 2 vols., Lond., 1885.

Strong, R.P., *Stitt's Diagnosis, Prevention and Treatment of Tropical Diseases*, Lond., 1945.

Tabler, E.C., *The Far Interior*, C.T., 1955.

Walker, K., *The Story of Medicine*, Lond., 1954.

Watson, Sir Malcolm, *African Highway*, Lond., 1953.

West, R., *Brazza of the Congo*, Lond., 1972.

Wilcocks, C., *Aspects of Medical Investigation in Africa*, Lond., 1942.

Wilson, C.M., *Ambassadors in White*, N.Y., 1942.

Wood, C., (ed.), *Tropical Medicine from Romance to Reality*, Lond., 1978.

Woodruff, A.W., *Medicine in the Tropics*, Lond., 1974.

Wostenholm, G., & O'Connor, M., (eds), *Man and Africa*, Ciba. 1965.

Zinsser, H., *Rats, Lice and History*, Boston, 1935.

Index